Praise for Brad's Work

"Brad has become a Bodhisattva who goes back into the perils he left behind to show others the way out. Brad can help you navigate the way to truth, love, and healing."
—ALICE WALKER,
PULITZER PRIZE–WINNING AUTHOR OF
THE COLOR PURPLE

JUST
10 LBS.

ALSO BY BRAD LAMM

How to Change Someone You Love: Four Steps to Help You Help Them

How to Help the One You Love: A New Way to Intervene and Stop Someone from Self-Destructing

JUST 10 LBS.

Easy Steps to Weighing
What You Want
(Finally)

BRAD LAMM

HAY HOUSE, INC.
Carlsbad, California • New York City
London • Sydney • Johannesburg
Vancouver • Hong Kong • New Delhi

Published and distributed in the United States by: Hay House, Inc.: www.hayhouse.com •
Published and distributed in Australia by: Hay House Australia Pty. Ltd.: www.hayhouse
.com.au • *Published and distributed in the United Kingdom by:* Hay House UK, Ltd.: www
.hayhouse.co.uk • *Published and distributed in the Republic of South Africa by:* Hay House
SA (Pty), Ltd.: www.hayhouse.co.za • *Distributed in Canada by:* Raincoast: www.raincoast
.com • *Published in India by:* Hay House Publishers India: www.hayhouse.co.in

Design: Celia Fuller

Author's Note: Case study names and locations have been changed.

Library of Congress Cataloging-in-Publication Data

Lamm, Brad.
  Just 10 lbs. : easy steps to weighing what you want (finally) / Brad Lamm.
     p. cm.
  ISBN 978-1-4019-3179-7 (hardcover : alk. paper) 1. Weight loss--Psychological aspects.. 2. Reducing exercises. 3. Behavior modification. 4. Obesity--Psychological aspects. I. Title. II. Title: Just ten pounds.
  RM222.2.L338 2011
  613.2'5--dc22
                          2011002395

Tradepaper ISBN: 978-1-4019-3185-8
Digital ISBN: 978-1-4019-3180-3

15 14 13 12   5 4 3 2
1st edition, January 2011
2nd edition, January 2012

Printed in the United States of America

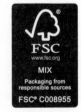

To coming out of your emotional-eating closet and discovering why you overeat.

We will take these steps together.

Nothing short of freedom awaits.

Contents

Acknowledgments

This book began as a broad idea that our *Dr. OZ* audience could live better and longer by losing just ten pounds at a time. Truth is, if we eat differently and resolve the emotional levers we pull to feed something other than physical hunger, we can change the world. *Just 10 Lbs.* is a reflection of Dr. Oz's commitment to helping people find their voice in making lifestyle choices. To Mehmet Oz, you inspire me to do more, to not just inform but inspire others!

Were it not for my *Dr. OZ Show* Executive Producer Mindy Borman, this book would not be in your hands. Mindy ushered the very concept each step of the way. Thank you, thank you, thank you. It's even sweeter since we go way, way back. So through history, love, and change, we made *Just 10 Lbs.* come to life.

Also at *The Dr. OZ Show,* Terence Noonan, Tim Sullivan, and Tina Tung have been amazing partners in time—helping me flesh out the big ideas in *Just 10 Lbs.* in the effort to help folks on the other side of their TV live lighter and better. Amazing work.

To all the folks I have helped find change, healing, and wholeness— I got something great in return: purpose.

To Maggie Greenwood-Robinson, my heartfelt thanks. You are rich and good and bright. I am so grateful you're on my team. To Todd Schuster, thanks for being more than an agent; you are a true friend and creative partner. To Patty Gift and everyone at Hay House, thanks for the opportunity to bring my work to millions. Louise Hay, you have my admiration and love. In the early 1990s, when New York City was breaking from the first wave of the AIDS epidemic, when compassion was rare (and hope even rarer), you gave love in ways that reverberate still.

There are so many loved ones who helped along the way. Thanks to each: Jerry, Scott, Fabio, Ken, Alfredo, Cathay, Fabrice, Javier, and Corey. And to my husband, Scott, and our family—we're writing the rules, sweetheart.

Bryant Stiney and Lisa Roberts-Lehan. You inspire me to move more and eat great. Thanks for your time, talent, friendship, and inspiration in making *Just 10 Lbs.*

To all of you who desire a life of dreams come true, jump into *Just 10 Lbs.* with me. We are how we eat.

Foreword

BY MEHMET OZ, M.D.

O besity is proving to be the great epidemic of our time. At its simplest, it is the result of too many calories consumed combined with too little exercise. The office of the U.S. surgeon general reports that 61 percent of Americans are obese and the cost to treat them is well above $100 billion a year. Sadly, obesity directly results in over 300,000 unnecessary deaths annually. Further, Americans who are obese have a 50 to 100 percent higher risk of death compared with those who live at a healthy weight. This is unacceptable and so very preventable, and yet so many of us feel powerless as we watch this epidemic spiral out of control in our own lives and in the lives of our friends, families, and communities. We see our loved ones struggle and wonder, *What can I do to help*?

What's needed is an easy-to-follow action plan for losing weight and addressing the underlying reasons why we overeat in the first place, then get sick as a result. When Brad Lamm first shared with me the idea of "Mend, Move, and Maintain," it immediately struck me as a powerful way for us to make—and keep—the lifestyle changes we most need to stay at a healthy weight. Mend your soul. Move your body. And maintain a healthy weight. It's that easy.

I am committed, as a doctor and father, husband and friend, to use what influence I have to highlight how, working together, we can end our nationwide crisis of obesity. My desire is simple:

that we start today—not waiting for another birthday or holiday to pass—and get down to business immediately.

For many who are thin, it's easy to look at a fat friend or neighbor and wonder, *Why don't they just stop overeating?* The causes of obesity are varied. I talked with my wife, Lisa, to see what she finds challenging regarding her relationship with food. She said it inevitably comes back to one thing: emotional eating.

So, I asked my friend Brad Lamm, a board-registered interventionist, the following question: what makes emotionally linked habits so hard to break, even in the face of mounting evidence that we are dying pound by pound and robbing ourselves and our families of loving relationships? His answer made a lot of sense to me: "I used to celebrate something special, or commiserate about something hurtful, by eating. I built that habit over years; and when I needed to change, it was hard, tough work for a time." Brad explained how the issue for so many Americans is fueled by the need to resolve conflicted feelings instead of using food to "numb out and suppress these feelings. In those cases, instead of feeding the body's needs, we're feeding the underlying, unsatisfied emotional needs." I think he's right—and therefore I see the deep importance and power of his simple, loving approach. Brad helps people get real results by showing them how to (a) eat differently, (b) clean house emotionally, and (c) help other folks they love to change their food habits, too.

As a practicing surgeon who performs more than 100 heart operations each year, I very much want you to focus on the impact that unhealthy eating habits and weight gain can and will have on your health, quality of life, and life expectancy. When I say "life expectancy," yes, I mean how long you can live a full, robust life. But I also mean what you wake up every day *expecting of yourself and your life*—what you think you can accomplish in the precious remaining years you have on this good earth.

We've all heard the saying that every cigarette you smoke takes 6 minutes off your life—actually, current research from the University of Bristol puts the number closer to 11 minutes. But did you know that each 10 pounds over your healthy weight robs you of precious time, too?

Consider the following fundamental truth at the center of this book: *Losing just 10 pounds will significantly decrease your risk for heart attack, stroke, hypertension, and diabetes.* Then, too, losing those 10 pounds will also likely increase your self-esteem, enhance your sex life, improve the way your clothes fit, and elevate your general outlook on life. When we decided to make *Just 10 Lbs.* the core initiative of season two of *The Dr. OZ Show,* I felt very pleased and proud because while the goal of losing only 10 pounds is small and reasonable enough for almost anyone to attain, the personal and wider social impact of making this change can be tremendous.

Just 10 Lbs. offers a jump start for lasting personal transformation. It is based on proven medical science, and I have seen with my own eyes just how effective Brad and his program can be.

As Brad will tell you himself, if anyone needed to change, it was him. In years past, he was addicted to alcohol, illegal drugs, food, and tobacco. Yet here he is today, helping others, shining light on pathways to positive change.

As I try to convey in the work I do regularly on *The Dr. OZ Show*, I am passionate about helping you lead the charge, to take control once again, to advocate for your own health and body. I encourage you to use the book you're holding in your hands to launch and stick with this very mission. Follow the steps Brad outlines in these pages—and keep your focus on losing those critical first 10 pounds. As you do, I know you'll start a new dialogue with yourself about food and about who you are, why you're here, and what you're going to contribute to others going forward. I am confident that you will begin to love yourself differently, especially through the way you feed and nourish your most precious of possessions: YOU!

I have no vested interest in this book—I'm not profiting off it in any way, but I hope you read *Just 10 Lbs.* simply because it will change the way you think and *feel* about food. Brad's 10-step plan will help you to identify your eating style, modify your eating habits, get your body moving, and love yourself more (as I always say, *you can't love yourself too much!*). As you move into a whole new physical and emotional place in your life, you can make brilliant plans for your future and look forward to getting closer to all of the goals you have for yourself. You may soon become a role model to your family, friends, and co-workers—even your entire community.

Recently Brad and I were on the stage together in Chicago at the Dr. OZ Health Fair to talk with a crowd of thousands, and the audience responded enthusiastically. As Brad talked with the crowd to inspire them to begin change in that moment, they answered affirmatively to his question: "Who is ready to begin to change and take the *Just 10* Pledge?!"

The crowd hollered out, in hope and desire: "ME!"

Brad knows, as do I, that it won't be easy at first. But be comforted by the fact that you are not alone. I am here by your side and so, too, are the thousands of people nationwide joining our mission. Let yourself join the *Just 10* movement. Do so and you'll soon see your body reduce while your spirit soars.

To feeling great and living your healthiest life.

— DR. MEHMET OZ

Say Good-bye to Just 10 Pounds in 30 Days

You're cleaning out your attic and you find a dusty lamp with a lid on the top. Although it looks to be about 1,000 years old, there's a magical glow around it, an aura. You immediately recognize it for what it is: a genie's lamp. You look around for a clean place to sit down—you, your lamp, and your future that just became brighter than a bucket of sunshine. Your heart pounds as you remove the lid, rub the lamp, and wait for something magical to occur. For a few seconds, nothing happens; and you start peeking around from side to side, hoping no one has noticed the biggest fool in the world.

Just then, a huge cloud of smoke spews from the lamp, spitting out your own personal genie. He's about 9 feet tall, smells like mothballs, and looks a lot like Mr. Clean. He is about to grant you three wishes.

A recent poll of genies revealed that everyone who is granted three wishes uses one for becoming thin. Wanting to be thinner is one of those givens, like the fact that we all want to win the lottery; look like Halle Berry, Cindy Crawford, or George Clooney; and get a television set so enormous the neighbors can see what we're watching. People who don't want to better their bodies a tiny bit simply don't exist. Rub. Poof. Wish. Voilà? If only.

I'm not your personal genie. I'm someone just like you. I used to have a food problem that sent my weight up and down so many times I could have passed for a seesaw. I can't grant you three wishes, but making your dreams a reality is what I'm all about. I can help you discover how to weigh what you want, stop hating yourself every time a piece of candy or a chunk of chocolate crosses your lips, and be at peace with your body.

Welcome to *Just 10 Lbs.*

The goals of this book are simple:

- Lose 10 pounds in 30 days by following the 10 steps in this book. Each step tackles a different aspect of weight loss, from nutrition to spiritual support. Do the steps and losing weight will feel almost effortless, because it's a way of living, not a way of losing (weight).

- Reclaim the power and emotions you've handed over to the food and renounce your food fight.

- Open up the emotional blockages that clutter your path to living your life to its glorious potential.

- Learn to eat normally and live at a healthy weight.

- Create a lifestyle that emphasizes the mind, body, emotions, relationships, and, most important, your spirit.

Just 10 Lbs. offers a sustainable approach to normalizing your weight and stopping destructive eating habits. It is built around restoring a positive, loving relationship with yourself—one of the most overlooked factors in weight management. It's really a spiritual diet book.

You see, no matter why you overeat, I know that food is not your only problem. This statement may surprise you. But I've learned through my own experience and through my work as an interventionist, dealing with clients with food issues, emotional problems, addictions, and other disorders, that losing weight is not just about dieting, doing push-ups, crunching out thousands of sit-ups, or running on a treadmill. It's primarily about your relationship with yourself. Weighing what you want starts with you—the "you" between your ears more than the "you" under your clothes. If you're stuck in a self-loathing mind-set, or your eating is out of control, then it's very hard to do something good for yourself or treat yourself well. Those three pounds of gray matter between your ears (that's about what your brain weighs) represent the key!

So, why just 10 pounds? Many of us think big—way too big—when it comes to losing weight, working out, and eating better. Once we're in major overhaul mode, we plot dramatic self-improvement campaigns with jumbo goals like losing 30, 50, or 100 pounds or more. The problem with such ambition, of course, is the potential for failure. Obsessing over a big loss can be overwhelming. And it may keep you from sticking to your weight-loss program. So I want you to forget the big weight-loss numbers for now. Let's focus on just 10. It's a winning strategy.

In fact, studies conducted at the University of Pennsylvania School of Medicine have shown that obese men and women who set a more modest goal of losing just 5 to 10 percent of their body weight are more likely to succeed than those who set more extreme goals.

Long-term goals alone—for instance, wanting to go down three dress sizes before bathing-suit season or wanting to lose 20 pounds in two weeks—fail to motivate healthy behavior because they are too distant to inspire you to make smart choices dozens of times a day. Short-term goals are doable, while long-term goals can be a fantasy. Say you weigh 175 and want to trim down to 140. If all you think about is 140, it minimizes the tremendous accomplishment of losing 10 pounds, because it's "only" 10 pounds. Having small, achievable goals creates a positive feedback loop that nurtures your resolve and fuels your internal motivation.

When we launch into a weight-loss program, our motivations are most commonly things like improving appearance, having more energy or better self-esteem, and other readily noticeable factors. And that's all great—because I'm sure you want to rock in your skinny jeans again. But there are some pretty impressive health benefits you gain by losing just 10 pounds. Let's take a look.

In a large National Institutes of Health clinical trial called the Diabetes Prevention program, more than 3,000 overweight people with impaired glucose tolerance (a prediabetic condition) were randomly assigned to a placebo group, a drug group, or a lifestyle intervention group (with low-fat diet, 30 minutes of daily exercise, and behavior modification). On average, the intervention group lost 5 to 7 percent of their body weight (11 pounds to 15 pounds) and reduced their risk of type 2 diabetes by 58 percent, significantly more than those on oral medication.

In the second phase of a National Institutes of Health study called the Trials of Hypertension Prevention, overweight people were randomly assigned to weight-loss intervention. Those who lost as few as 10 pounds over six months—and kept it off for two years—experienced significant reductions in blood pressure and fewer subsequent diagnoses of high blood pressure than those who didn't lose weight.

So, just 10 pounds? You may be rewarded with some big health payoffs! It doesn't look as insignificant now, does it?

Now is as good a time as any to introduce myself. I am a board-registered interventionist and addiction specialist. I am also a former addict and a compulsive overeater. I now devote my life to helping others, because I know firsthand what it takes to break the cycle of self-abuse.

I grew up in a large, loving home in Eugene, Oregon, the youngest of four boys of a minister. Food was an important part of my home life for as long as I can remember. We had a large garden out back in which my dad and I planted, tended, and harvested the bulk of our fruits and vegetables. My first job was the "little green grocer" in our own backyard. I bagged and sold the produce from a red wagon door-to-door to help out with our family finances. Looking back, I loved my young life, which now seems as idyllic as a *My Three Sons* episode, but with a mother, Nancy, and an extra son—me.

My first encounter with weight issues occurred when, as a child, I found my mother weighing carrots on a little scale before dinner. "Mom, what are you doing?" I asked. Weighing carrots, to me, seemed like a very strange thing to do.

"I'm overweight," she told me. "I'm on a diet, and I have to lose weight." Now you have to know that my mother was a lovely young woman. But all she could think about was how fat she was. She turned into a compulsive yo-yo dieter, and that's how she lived.

And so, I grew up in a family where there was pressure to diet. Everyone gained weight and everyone dieted. Everybody, except for one of my brothers, was heavy at one time or another. Every meal in our family was a binge, with portions that were three times the norm.

My mom led our diet craziness. She would take 15 off, and then pack on 20. Trim 25 with the help of Jenny Craig, only to yo-yo back up, with interest. She'd try pills and powders. She gulped Ayds diet candy like, well, candy. Remember those? (The emergence of AIDS killed the brand's popularity, and it was taken off the market.) She battled her weight, up and down, here and there, into one fad diet after another for her entire life. All my momma could do was worry about how fat she was and how she could get skinny. Food was her obsession.

As a family, we thinned, expanded, binged, and climbed back on the wagon, depending on where Mom was with her food at a given time. Our family started and stopped more diets than I can remember. I don't blame or shame her for this. It was just part of our story.

Mom's cholesterol got dangerously high, too—a serious problem that sadly cost her the life she loved. Three years ago, while picking flowers in the rose garden in the Quaker retirement village where she and Dad lived, Mom suffered a massive stroke. She has never recovered—the left lobe of her brain literally died—and her condition has been a blow to our family. The mom we loved, the grandma we hoped the kids would enjoy for decades to come, was without half her brain.

Looking back, I mimicked my mom's eating and dieting habits while growing up. As a kid, I started eating in secret, hiding frozen spritz cookies and other goodies in my sweatshirt for the walk to my bedroom, where I would console myself or celebrate a triumph. Joy. Comfort. Celebration. Pain. Hunger. I ate for all those reasons, and more.

At college, my food intake went up and down by turns. I felt fat, pathetic, and self-conscious. I would gain and lose the same 20 pounds I'd been struggling to keep off since I was a teen. Dorm food zipped it right back on. It seemed like I was heavier than everyone I hung out with, and I started to hate myself for being unable to lose weight again.

Then my thin-as-a-rail friend Valerie showed me how to "get rid of it" by purging. Throw it up. Gross, right? But that was my remedy—don't keep the enemy down. Unhealthy and self-destructive as it was, that was what my best thinking got me. Soon, I was preoccupied with bingeing and purging—and I was anything but in control. I was in the grips of an upside-down relationship with food, and it was called bulimia.

I struggled with bulimia and compulsive binge eating for many years, but I didn't look thin enough or sick enough for anyone (including me) to think I needed help. "You've lost weight," I would hear countless times, though friends would stay silent when I'd go from a size 30 waist back to a 35. I just kept my food fight to myself, year after year and tragedy after triumph.

But that's not all. I started drinking alcohol as a kid; I liked the way it made me feel. Alcohol led to recreational drugs, lots of them. Food was a balm, too; I ate to soothe myself.

In 2001, I was pushing 197 pounds at around 5 foot 9. I'd start my day with a 32-ounce Dr. Pepper from 7-Eleven. That's approximately 28 ounces of soda and 4 ounces of ice, clocking in at a brain-changing jolt of 128 grams of sugar and 512 calories in one shot. By the time summer 2002 rolled around, I had added a six-pack of Red Bull per day, boosting my sugar intake by an additional 132 grams per day. I was wired and on fire from my food and drink choices.

The sugar, the food, the alcohol—it all made me fat. I was desperate to stay trim and avoid those "10 pounds" they say being on television adds (I worked in television for many years). I smoked to control my appetite and keep the weight off. I binged and purged. If it wasn't one thing . . . it was another!

I hated myself and my lack of self-control. No matter how hard I tried, I always ended up right back where I started: in the drugs, the alcohol, the nicotine, the sugar, and the food. I was self-medicating with everything I could get my hands on.

I'd look in the mirror and think, *What happened?* I had the résumé of a model citizen, not a common drunk or addict. Hometown: Eugene, Oregon. Occupation: weather anchor. Parents: beloved minister and devoted mother, both of whom raised me in an alcohol-free home with lots of love.

In other words, nice person, from a decent middle-class family. Why couldn't I beat my addictions? Of course, there is no simple answer. Trying to describe the process of becoming an addict is like trying to describe space. It's too big and mysterious and pervasive to be defined. All you know is that you can't live without your vice(s).

I went through countless detoxes and even more diets to get cleaned up. But I didn't keep the postdetox or postdiet promises. Active addicts try, and active addicts fail. That's how it works. I made the promises, and I really did try to keep them. But I kept rationalizing the third drink or the fourth or fifth, or the box of doughnuts or the package of chocolate chip cookies. *Just today. Bad day. I deserve a reward,* I told myself. *I'll stop tomorrow.*

I hated myself into multiple, life-threatening addictions that could have robbed me of the chance to share my story with you. Sickened, drained, unable to feel—it was perpetual numbness. No sadness, no happiness, no highs, no lows. Nothing. This is why addictions are so difficult to kick. My pleasure receptors were so fried that my brain no longer had the ability to feel any pleasure on its own. When you're that addicted, you're so depressed that you just want to get high, again and again.

All told, I spent 20 years living in addiction. But through the help of friends and therapists, I got into rehab for one last time. Recovery was rough, tough going. I spent hours tracing my relapse history and building a timeline of progression, identifying many of the feelings and thoughts that led to each setback. One therapist told me, "Brad, you have a choice. You can begin to love yourself today or you can die from all this."

Whoa. My struggles were causing me emotional pain, but I didn't think they could kill me. I didn't want to die. But I didn't even like myself anymore. How was I going to achieve self-love?

There weren't any infomercials selling me a quick, easy way to do that. But when I was 34 years old, I finally broke free from my self-defeating, life-robbing behavior. I did it through intense work and many of the steps you'll learn on these pages.

Your story might be different, but I'm sure at one time or another you've found yourself reaching for a bag of chips or a pint of ice cream without realizing what you're doing. Sometimes it's for no reason other than sheer boredom. Other times you're on auto-pilot. You grab some cookies when really you're looking for a way to kill time, or you snag a box of this or that to eat instead of thinking about what's eating you. Other times it may be to soothe yourself or detour around uncomfortable feelings. To some degree, we all do this. If you're gaining weight because of it, or you can't stop eating certain foods, or eating is taking the place of building closer connections with the people in your life, then it's a sign that something is wrong.

After many years helping thousands of people change, and after combating and healing my own up-and-down relationship with food and eating, I have come to a vital truth around food and weight—a truth that will help you, as it helped me, finally weigh what you want and find peace with food.

Here is that truth: When you change your relationship with yourself—when you truly begin to love yourself—you will change your relationship with food, too. You will break the cycles of over-eating, and you will be more likely to *stay* at your healthy weight.

I used to regret the time I wasted being unhappy with my body and being self-destructive. Now I use my history and path to teach and help others. I don't want you to waste another second. My hope is that *Just 10 Lbs.* will encourage you to find happiness and peace with yourself. I will teach you how to let go of a self-destructive, restrictive relationship with food. It may feel like I'm helping you pry it loose from your grip, but you'll make peace with food and with your body if you'll let me show you how. You'll learn about inviting into your life the experience of eating wholesome foods and doing so in a meditative, loving way with your friends and family, rather than squirreling yourself away to eat crap in isolation.

You'll discover how to heal yourself emotionally and spiritually, and bring that power and connective soothing force to others, as a parent does to a child.

I know that each day, I wake up with a choice, and by choosing not to binge eat, or drink alcohol, or do drugs, just for that day, I am a better son, friend, husband, and colleague. I choose to enjoy the gifts that come from a healthy life, a loving relationship with my family, the ability to help others through my work, and a strong faith.

As an interventionist, I have had the privilege of working with people from all walks of life, with many different kinds of struggles. I have been startled and concerned by how many people and families are struggling with weight and food problems. It was overwhelming, and I knew in my heart that I had to devote a special area of my work to weight management.

Some people say, "If you haven't walked in my shoes, you don't know." Well, I know. I can empathize with what you're feeling because I have been there myself.

Through solving my own weight and food problems, I discovered a few things. I learned how losing weight and freeing myself from a food *addiction* changed both my life and how I viewed myself. It made me happier, more confident, and successful. I wanted to help other people *not* go through the things I had to experience. I wanted to make a difference to them.

Thus, I became an interventionist on a mission. It is now my dream that people of all ages who struggle with this problem don't have to face it alone, and that they can overcome unhealthy lifestyle habits if they have the right tools.

Being overweight and having food issues have multiple causes, and thus must be approached from multiple angles. Food, exercise, body image, emotional healing, spiritual power, and more—all of these are the very same techniques that led to my own change. In my work, I use a 10-step program that anyone can use to lose weight, no matter how many times they have failed in the past.

Since developing this 10-step program, I've witnessed the joy, surprise, and relief of my clients as they learn that losing weight my way doesn't have to be a frustrating, angst-ridden chore. It can be positive and full of self-discovery. Getting this kind of feedback affected me profoundly. It lit a fire under me. I understood how the work I was doing was unique and powerful.

These steps will help you, as they helped me. Here are some coming attractions.

Step 1: Live the Love-Centered Diet

For many people, food is like a drug, which could explain why many of us just can't stop bingeing, particularly on junk food. The Love-Centered Diet simplifies your eating and gives your body a 30-day break from refined flour, sugar, and junk food. You'll shed excess fluid, gain more energy, improve your digestion, and of course, begin to lose weight. I call this food plan the "Love-Centered Diet" because it focuses on foods that "love" your body: pure, natural foods, all bursting with nutrients that add to your health and well-being. Your eating style counts, too. You'll learn how to eat in a less hectic or tense atmosphere, without reacting to your emotions or outside influences, and enjoy your food by paying attention to all your senses.

Step 2: Start a Moving Meditation

Learn how to go beyond the "sweat mentality" of exercise and experience physical activity in a whole new way: as a "moving meditation." This involves exercising mindfully, instead of think-ing about reps, sets, pace, or steps—or what's for dinner. A moving meditation can involve any form of activity, from yoga to swim-ming to lifting weights. It teaches you to reflect on your inside self. The benefits can range from reduced stress to communion with the divine.

Step 3: Develop a Daily Practice

What would it take for you to feel less stressed and more in control of your food and well-being all day long? Just 10 minutes in the morning, with what I call a "daily practice." It's an easy way to find calm and set the tone you want for the day ahead.

Step 4: Appreciate Your Body

Beating yourself up about how big your belly looks in that swimsuit or how much skinnier your sister is may seem like powerful motivation to lose weight. But, in fact, negative body-image thoughts like these can have the opposite effect, causing you to gain extra pounds. The reason: research suggests that learning to accept and, yes, even to love your body just the way it is can actually help you lose weight. Step 4 shows you how to reverse those negative mind-sets for good—and reap the slimming benefits.

Step 5: Love Yourself Thin

Loving yourself is the most overlooked factor in weight management. Lack of self-love while simmering in fear leads to mindless, unhealthy eating—and can take the form of overweight and obesity. If you're stuck in a self-loathing mind-set, or your eating is out of control, then it's very hard to do something good for yourself, or treat yourself well. In this step, I will teach you how to love yourself—perhaps for the first time ever—through a series of thought-provoking questions that will help you make healthier choices and take responsibility for your life.

Step 6: Maintain Loving Connections

People who lose weight—and keep it off—generally have help. Proof: in one recent study, the men and women who participated in a structured weight-loss program that included weekly group support lost more weight and did a better job of keeping it off for two years than the people who lacked group support. Step 6 shows you how to build the type of support and accountability that will get you through the days when you don't want to keep at it. At the end of your rope is hope (and help).

Step 7: Eliminate Excuses

We all tell ourselves stories that explain—or make excuses for—how we've come to be the way we are, or why we act the way we do. The trick is to create a new narrative, one that reflects your goals, and why and how you can effect the change you're aiming for. In this step, I'll show you how to strategize around typical excuses like "I don't have time to exercise" or "I have a slow metabolism" and get on track for good.

Step 8: Examine Your Battleground Beliefs

Your battleground beliefs are the thoughts running through your head 24/7. These opinions, which are formed in childhood, are often subconscious; but we filter everything through them, from the way we see ourselves in the mirror to an offhand comment a friend makes. So if one of your battleground beliefs is "I'm a failure because I can't stick to a diet," experiences that support that statement (you keep failing on diets) often follow, while those that seem to contradict it (you exercise three times a week) are simply discounted. Step 8 helps you adjust your outlook by forming positive beliefs you'd like to have, then imprinting them in your mind so that you're more in control of your life.

Step 9: Connect with Higher-Source Thinking

How we approach life and spirituality contributes to our overall well-being. People who tap into their spiritual side have a positive self-image, a sense of purpose in life, and better health than those who don't, according to a growing body of research. Spirituality—and I use that term very broadly—reminds us that life may have greater meaning, so we don't dwell so much on the little things. Step 9 shows you how to dial into the bigger picture with some simple practices that will help you meet your *Just 10* goal.

Step 10: Pay It Forward

Everyone is looking for the magical answer on how to keep weight off once you've lost it—and there are many effective solutions. In this 10th and final step, I'll give you what I believe to be the ultimate answer: you've got to pay it forward. This is the powerful helping-others step, and it starts with your friends and family. My change spread to my own family, and we've now lost more than 200 pounds. I've found that the best antidote to backsliding is finding someone who is in need with whom I can share my energy, love, and attention. When you bring a little fresh air into someone's life, expect some of that refreshing breeze to blow back your way.

These, then, are the steps to weighing what you want. They are easy to follow and will change your life if you work with them in the right way. You will need only a few tools to help you get as much out of this program as possible. As you go through the steps, I ask you to reflect on many different aspects of your life. This reflection will take the form of journaling, so before you begin, either buy a nice journal or go to *JUST10Challenge.com* and download the *Just 10 Workbook*. This workbook has not only ample space for journaling but also additional exercises and materials to help you go deeper into this process. So let's jump right in and get started.

CHAPTER ONE

STEP
1

Live the Love-
Centered Diet

oo often, we take our physical bodies for granted. We fill
them with wholly unsuitable foods in wholly unsuitable
amounts. We punish our bodies by neglecting their needs,
usually until it's too late and we're forced into a different way of
life because of poor health, rickety self-esteem, or yet another set
of clothes we've outgrown.

Once I got "clean and lean," I started to see the human body for
what it really is: an amazing and intelligent creation that we need
to love and respect. I had this wonderful, capable body, but I was
wasting it in a gradual decline at a young age! I wanted to feel more
alive and more energetic. I wanted a healthier heart, thicker hair,
and stronger muscles. I wanted stamina in life and the bedroom. I
knew the only way to achieve those things on the outside depended
almost entirely on what I put in the inside. I knew I had to give my
body more love.

One of the best ways to do this is through food—natural,
wholesome foods, not artery-clogging junk or sugary foods that
pack on weight. Why is this important? Because your body uses
pure, natural food much more efficiently than it uses processed,
chemical-laden food, such as refined cereals; commercially baked

goods; or fat-, sugar-, and additive-loaded snacks—or even the unhealthy fat-free foods that have jacked-up sugar content. Pure food is bursting with quality nutrition and is put to use in building and healing the body.

And so, Step 1 is about taking care of and loving your body with nutritious food—which is why I call my food plan the Love-Centered Diet.

There are actually two parts to the Love-Centered Diet.

First, you'll learn how to eat according to your personal style (there are six styles). Many of us are inclined to eat in a great rush or in response to negative emotions, cravings, or deeply ingrained bad habits. Those are ruts we've got to get out of to get our weight under control. This part of Step 1 gets your head in the game by giving you strategies that match your personal style of eating.

Second, you'll follow the Love-Centered food plan. It helps you transition from eating the typical American meat-heavy, sugar-laden, low-fiber fare to consuming naturally delicious, slimming, body-honoring foods. This is a sensible diet that gets results. Expect to lose weight right away, and up to two pounds for each additional week that you stay with the plan. My brother Scott lost 16 pounds the first month on the plan, and I've had clients lose that and more. The point is, you eat differently and fall into the plan we'll work on together, and the weight will fall off. Stick with it 30 days and you'll be 10 pounds lighter—or more.

Also, on the Love-Centered Diet, you'll *feel* better, and you'll be more at peace with yourself. As you follow this plan, try to remember to love yourself—body and mind—for the whole, multifaceted person you are. You're not just a body, but when you love your body for what it is, rather than hate it for what it's not, you'll take care of it—and the pounds will come off effortlessly.

You Are How You Eat

You've heard the expression "You are what you eat." Well, it's not altogether true. You are also *how* you eat. Understanding this is very important to improving your diet, restoring a healthy balance to your body, and arriving at your healthy weight.

As you've probably gathered, to shed 10 pounds, we're not just going to change what we eat; we've got to change *how* we eat. Nobody talks about this. Everyone talks about giving up fries, Big Macs, and cheesecakes. Or worse, they promise a Don't-Change-One-Thing-You-Eat diet as the next empty miracle. We will focus on how we eat—and trust me, the what will take care of itself.

Each of us eats differently. This is our eating style. Understanding this is important to weight loss because it gets your head in the game, shows you behavioral changes you need to make, and helps you become more aware of the taste and texture of your food. Every single pound will be a struggle to lose unless you eat according to your style.

If you can identify which of the six eating styles you have, you'll be able to understand how to deal with food and use it to honor your body. So any sound nutritional plan needs to include a reality check about your style of eating, as well as what you're eating.

On the next two pages you'll find a questionnaire to help you become your own mealtime detective. It will make you think about your eating habits and help you find out which eating style you are. There are no right and wrong answers—just guidelines to reveal clues about your personal eating style.

Read through the following statements, and check the ones that best apply to you. Be honest with yourself.

Section A

☐ As a child, I often received food as a reward for good behavior.
☐ As a child, I often received food to comfort me.
☐ I eat when I'm experiencing negative emotions.
☐ I eat when I'm happy or joyful.
☐ I tend to reward myself by eating out at restaurants.
☐ I eat when I'm bored.
☐ I sometimes feel guilty after eating.
☐ I have sometimes hidden my eating from my family and friends.
☐ My diet is filled with so-called "comfort foods" that act as a security blanket: macaroni and cheese, meatballs and gravy, grilled-cheese sandwiches, or cookies.
☐ When something goes wrong at work, I abandon my healthy diet and eat whatever I please.

Section B

☐ I eat at certain times of the day, even though I might not be hungry.
☐ Many of my family gatherings and celebrations center on food.
☐ I frequently supersize my meals or order large portions on purpose.
☐ I eat fast food for lunch because it is the easiest option.
☐ I am not aware of how many calories I might consume on a given day or at a given meal or snack.
☐ I usually can't remember everything I've eaten for the day.
☐ I nibble mostly out of habit.
☐ At times, I'm surprised by the amount of weight I've gained.
☐ I was required to clean my plate as a child.
☐ I'm a nighttime eater or a refrigerator raider.

Section C

☐ I sometimes continue to eat even after I feel full.
☐ I go off my diet easily at parties and social gatherings.
☐ Food advertising makes me hungry.
☐ I crave food at certain times of the day.
☐ If I smell food as I pass my favorite drive-through or bakery, I'm apt to succumb.
☐ *For women:* My appetite or eating changes according to my menstrual cycle.
☐ I often shop for groceries when I am hungry.
☐ I can't stick to my list when I'm grocery shopping.
☐ I have a sweet tooth.
☐ I have good intentions when I go to a restaurant but usually end up making less-healthy choices or overeat.

Section D

- [ ] I believe my life would improve if I lost weight.
- [ ] Embarrassment about my weight has kept me from doing something I want to do.
- [ ] I count nearly every calorie and every gram of fat, carbohydrate, and protein I put in my mouth.
- [ ] I consider myself well versed in nutrition.
- [ ] If I blow my diet at one meal, I figure I've blown my whole diet, and I go on a binge.
- [ ] I would do anything to meet my weight goal.
- [ ] I have sometimes avoided eating at restaurants or at parties for fear of falling off my diet.
- [ ] If I overeat, I make sure to go to the gym to work it off.
- [ ] I read nutritional labels.
- [ ] I tend to judge others by what they eat.

Section E

- [ ] I love to cook, read food magazines, and clip recipes.
- [ ] I do most of the food shopping in my household.
- [ ] I do most of the cooking in my household.
- [ ] I enjoy watching cooking shows on television.
- [ ] I love to try new foods and restaurants.
- [ ] I appreciate food and savor every nuance of every bite—the textures, aromas, and flavors.
- [ ] I don't hold back at restaurants. I clean my plate.
- [ ] I rarely deny myself any food.
- [ ] Celebrity chefs are my heroes.
- [ ] I love giving gifts of food.

Section F

- [ ] I eat in response to powerful cravings for sugary, salty, or fatty foods.
- [ ] I have specific food cravings that are hard to resist.
- [ ] My snack of choice is usually chocolate or something sweet.
- [ ] I sometimes wake up at night craving ice cream.
- [ ] Exercising makes me very hungry.
- [ ] I count on coffee and other caffeinated beverages to keep me going.
- [ ] I need a sugary pick-me-up most afternoons.
- [ ] I get obsessed over leftover cake or brownies and tend to eat them till they're gone.
- [ ] I've binged in front of the refrigerator.
- [ ] I've been told that I'm allergic to some foods.

Look over your answers. Wherever you have the most check marks, that is your eating style. Once you've identified your style, move on to the next section: Understand Your Style. It will give you style-based strategies and affirmations to help you lose your first 10 pounds. Could you be a combination of all these styles or a combination of a few of them? Definitely! I am a combo of A, C, D, and F. Put together, it spells nothing, but it means a lot.

If you are a combo, too, I suggest you read through the strategies for each style. Are there any in particular that resonate with you—that you think might be useful? If so, circle those and make them a part of your personal overall eating strategy. Information is power, and tagging your style or styles helps you build your understanding and take appropriate actions around food and eating.

Once you identify your eating style, consider the challenges and solutions, and then say the affirmation out loud. Speak it clearly and lovingly to yourself. Later in this program, we'll discuss the importance of a daily practice. I encourage you to include the affirmation(s) in your daily practice also. Weaving these words into your quiet time of reflection will help you reframe the way you feed yourself based on your eating style.

Understand Your Style

A. *The Emotional Eater*

CHALLENGES: To a great extent, we are all emotional eaters. It's baked into our culture. Early on, we learn to associate food with love. When a baby cries, the first thing a parent offers is breast milk or some other food. Using food for comfort is a normal, healthy impulse. And when it's only one of many ways you take care of yourself, eating something can be a very nice way to make yourself feel better.

But if you're gaining weight because of it, or you can't stop eating certain foods, or eating is taking the place of building closer connections with the people in your life, it's a sign that something is wrong. Eating might be an escape from uncomfortable emotions or a conflicting feeling.

For emotional eaters, food is closely linked to how you feel. Happiness is celebrated with food; and when things are going wrong, you console yourself with food. The problem here is that emotional eating never solves your problem. It just creates another one, with food.

JUST 10 **STRATEGIES:** For starters, keep a food journal—either in your personal journal or in your *Just 10 Workbook*—listing what you eat and how you were feeling when you ate it. This will identify what feelings trigger you to eat—and what need you're really feeding. You can then try to find ways to reduce that need. When I was upset and wanted to turn to food for comfort, I wrote in a journal. This helped me discover some things about my eating patterns, and you should look out for things like this also:

- **Boredom:** Studies show most emotional eating occurs between 7 P.M. and 10 P.M. Are you eating to fill time?

- **Stress:** Most of us don't look at why stress is in our lives. We just focus on controlling it, in this case, with food. Develop interesting hobbies that take your mind off of food, and relieve stress with exercise you enjoy. (Be sure to practice Step 2—see Chapter 2.)

- **Loneliness:** Do you use food to fill an emotional void in your life or in your relationships? This is a tough one to tackle, as many emotional eaters are more passive people who don't like confrontation. But if you're in a relationship that's not meeting your needs, you need to talk about it.

I'd like to see you beginning your day with a solid breakfast; cutting back on the amount of saturated fat; and filling your diet with fruits, vegetables, and other body-honoring food. Plan your meals each week, too.

I also suggest addressing the problem with therapy and guidance, so you can learn how to love yourself properly. This book is a good step. It will start you back on the path to loving yourself.

And when you really love yourself, there is no such thing as a weight problem.

YOUR AFFIRMATION: I am special. Because I am special, I choose food that makes me feel good physically and emotionally—body-honoring food that nourishes me and moves me toward a healthy weight. I understand my feelings and deal with them. No matter what is going on in my life, the right reaction is to bless my thoughts . . . bless those I have been blaming . . . and bless the circumstances that seem wrong. I continue blessing with all the power I possess. Peace, rest, and joy are mine.

B. The Habitual Eater

CHALLENGES: You have some wonderful strengths that can keep you at a healthy weight. You like routine and structure, for example, and you know how to eat right and exercise regularly. It's easy for you to establish good habits once you get started but tougher to make them stick when you hit emotional triggers.

What derails you—and many of us—are time constraints and responsibilities. They often keep you from following through with diet and exercise programs. You might have a full-time job that requires many extra hours, for example, or be a homemaker with family responsibilities and no time off.

Perhaps you've gotten in the habit of splurging by eating fast food for lunch because it's the easiest option, or maybe skipping lunch altogether and grazing on sugary or salt-laden snacks from vending machines. You rationalize by saying, "Eating fast food for just one meal won't hurt." Or maybe you're in a meeting that runs long, so you skip lunch "just this once" and rely on snacks later. Soon, "just this once" becomes your daily routine.

Some habitual eaters eat when they aren't hungry, simply because it is what they're used to doing. Your eating style keeps you from working up a normal appetite and eating on schedule. You think you're not eating a lot but then get ambushed by weight gain.

Maybe you've been known to unconsciously work your way through a tub of popcorn in the movie theater. At home, you might munch mindlessly while watching television without real-izing just how many empty calories you're eating. Perhaps you supersize your fast-food meals or go "fried" with an automatic yes, and you tend to eat everything on your plate whether you're full or not.

If you're in this category, you've lost weight before, so you know what success means. Your biggest challenge is to translate ini-tial lifestyle changes into permanent commitment.

JUST 10 STRATEGIES: We all know that we're creatures of habit. Each of us has formed habits around how we think about ourselves and how we react to life. Some of these ways add to our well-being, while others detract from it.

You want to add to your well-being, and you have the force of mind to do so. Follow your innate love of structure. Take an orga-nized approach to healthy eating. This might involve premeasured portions, predefined mealtimes, and even preset menus. Healthy meals don't happen by chance. They're planned.

Some journaling—either in your journal or your *Just 10 Workbook*—goes a long way, too. Make a habit of logging your meals. Write down everything you've eaten on one weekday and one weekend day. This will help you identify the hidden fats and empty calories you've been consuming. Eat it? Write it down. Period. No excuses. You know the drill. You can also use some of the additional exercises in your *Just 10 Workbook* to begin to do the deeper work. I promise it will offer release and relief.

Put the right tools in your nutrition toolbox. Stock your kitchen, cars, purses, and desk drawers with healthy snacks such as cut-up veggies, so when you reach for the nearest food, it will be doing your body the highest good. Remember, this isn't forever, it's for now, as you reboot and detox and retrain your need to feed.

We make our habits, then our habits make us. What will yours be?

YOUR AFFIRMATION: I'm grateful for my love of structure and routine. I use this strength to determine my living habits. I make healthy choices, because those choices determine the successes I achieve. Wise choices enliven me and encourage right action.

When I make a new, better choice, I change my attitudes, habits, and overall behavior for the better. My daily thinking and activity always follow a positive habitual course. My life is precious to me, and I am thankful for health and vitality.

C. The External Eater

CHALLENGES: The world we live in is incredibly beautiful and vibrant, with so many sights and sounds and paths to take. As we travel those paths, it's easy to get sidetracked by what we see along the way. Unfortunately, external cues to eat are all around us. Many of us overeat because we're triggered by these external cues: cupcakes in the display window, food advertising, restaurant offerings, smells of food wafting from eateries, and people or places that push food at us (even within our own home or office). All of this adds to the pressure or desire to overeat. Some of us—the external eaters—are more vulnerable than others.

JUST 10 **STRATEGIES:** When something triggers an urge to eat, try one of these strategies:

- **Create a distraction.** Call a friend, take a bath, read a book, listen to music. Another method of self-soothing (known by different names, including "tapping") involves rubbing a spot on your palm, or tapping a pencil on the counter, or even snapping your *Just 10* bracelet on your wrist (free from *ChangeInstitute.com*) to draw your attention away from the desire to binge. Distractions interrupt you and allow the craving to pass.

- **Snack right.** Very often a small amount of healthful food—some low-sugar fruit such as melon or berries, for example—can take away the pang.

- **Talk to yourself.** Ask: Am I really hungry? Is it really good for me to eat this food? Is this really what I want? What I need?

- **Create an "action" list.** When you discover a strategy that helps you cope with externally triggered eating, note it in your journal or your *Just 10 Workbook* and refer to it next time you find cheese-filled-crust pizza irresistible.

- **Keep the treats that make you binge out of your house.** That way, you won't come across them accidentally in the pantry, and it'll be harder to access them. You can't eat what's not there. If you really want cookies or chips, go to the store and buy a snack-size amount—just one small pack.

- **Change your route.** If you know that driving past the doughnut shop on the way to work will set you off, take a different route.

- **Take the edge off.** If you're going out to dinner with a bunch of friends or to a party and are concerned you'll overeat, have some natural high-fiber foods (like fresh fruits or raw vegetables) before you go. You'll be less likely to pig out.

YOUR AFFIRMATION: I say, "Enough is enough!" when I encounter a food-triggering situation. It has no more power to disrupt me, nor can it prevail against me. There is no shadow in my path, no barrier to my success, no situation too difficult to solve. Knowing this to be true, I take control of my life and circumstances.

D. The Critical Eater

CHALLENGES: You possess a lot of valuable knowledge about nutrition and health—knowledge you can access for weight control and healing. The problem is, though, that you tend to be obsessive about diets and dieting. You may have lots of self-imposed rules and regulations about what you eat. You're among those to whom dieting, to some degree, has become a religion. When dieting, you're considered "good"; when off the diet, you're "bad." This is a form of all-or-nothing thinking (you feel bad if you eat high-calorie food, believe you've blown it, and keep on eating), and critical eaters are masters at thinking in extremes.

Rather than living to eat, you eat to live. You don't particularly enjoy eating, but use food purely as a way to fuel your body. You keep count in your head of every calorie and every gram of fat, carbohydrate, and protein you put in your mouth. Perhaps you're an avid exerciser who will do anything to meet your weight goal. Maybe you're overweight and are desperately trying to drop the extra pounds. Whatever the case, you avoid eating at restaurants or at parties for fear of falling off the course of your diet plan.

While it's a good idea to know what's going into your body, a critical eater goes through mental anguish that shouldn't be associated with eating. Perhaps you act like a forensic scientist when it comes to what you eat, continually analyzing or forecasting doom and gloom over every morsel.

And you often push away family and friends when you avoid social gatherings that include meals. Nutritionally, low-calorie diets can also be hazardous if you deprive the body of essential nutrients.

JUST 10 **STRATEGIES:** I favor changing your ways completely. Throw away your food scale, calorie counters, and other measuring tools. Trust me: this can be a very freeing experience for you when you stop counting and weighing what you're eating.

- **Ease up on rigid food rules.** Concentrate less on what "bad" foods not to eat and more on getting enough fruits and vegetables.

  You might use food to gain a (false) sense of control over your life. You might give up dairy products because "it's good for your health." Don't do this. Try to eat normally, aiming for a variety of foods, focusing on healthy choices, but allowing all foods when your body wants them. The body needs dozens of different nutrients daily. That's something that you can only get by consuming lots of different kinds of foods.

- **Get over your food fears.** Many people in this group are afraid of food and think as soon as they come off their diet they will gain weight. Seeing a nutritionist can help you understand what makes a diet healthy.

- **Stop being so hard on yourself.** You've allowed shame and embarrassment to keep you from doing enjoyable activities. For example, you may not swim because you're afraid that other people will make fun of you in a swimsuit. Or perhaps you avoid taking a vacation that requires an airplane flight because you have to ask for a seat-belt extension or cannot fit into a seat.

  Women are tougher on themselves than men, so I have another suggestion. Why don't you join a women-only health club? You might feel more comfortable. Having some support will give you more body confidence, too. And the exercise will help you love your body more. Write in your journal or *Just 10 Workbook* about how you treat yourself and how you experience your feelings. This will help you identify patterns of behavior and emotion that could be getting in the way of your progress.

- **Jettison the all-or-nothing thinking (thinking about yourself in extremes).** Thoughts are creative. The character of your thoughts determines what they create. If you think of yourself as healthy and strong, your body takes actions to make it so.

  All-or-nothing thinking creates problems when one less-healthy choice in the day leads you to think "I've blown it now," so you spend the rest of the day practicing unhealthy behavior that you could have avoided. When you're on your diet, you're "being good," and when you lose that willpower, you slip over into "being bad," which often leads to unrestrained eating. There's no middle ground; you're totally in, or totally out of control.

  All-or-nothing thinking also forms the basis for perfectionism. It causes you to fear any mistake or imperfection, because you then will see yourself as a total loser. If you try to bend your life experiences into absolute or extreme categories, you will be constantly depressed whenever your expectations and perceptions do not conform to reality. Of course, you're not perfect, but you are a wonderful person. So, give yourself a break! And if you fall off the beam, "restart" your day at any time—don't allow a whole day to be lost to defeatist thinking.

- **Develop more realistic thinking.** An example of a realistic focus is "I can exercise and lose weight, but it takes time and hard work to reach my goals." Practice daily discipline in thought training and you'll get closer to your goals. Each day, think less of that which is destructive and more of that which produces health and success.

YOUR AFFIRMATION: I love my body. I feed it with a variety of body-honoring foods. I look and feel my best. I feed my mind with strong, positive, life-radiating ideas. How wonderful to know that I have the power to change my thoughts and attitudes, and thus to change the circumstances in which I find myself. I restart my day at any point. No matter what occupied my mind last year, last week, yesterday, or even a few moments ago, I have the power to adopt new and healthy attitudes, which produce good, and oftentimes miraculous, results.

E. The Sensual Eater

CHALLENGES: You appreciate food and relish every bite. You're a bit of a thrill seeker, always on the lookout for meals more complex and intriguing than your last. That usually means that you don't hold back. You wolf down every last bite of your pasta with lobster sauce and capers. You ask for extra herbed butter for your basket of rolls. It *is* fun being you when it comes to food!

To be honest, I really wish there were more people like you. Many people are so busy with work and/or family responsibilities that they just don't feel that they have the time to prepare and enjoy their food. Instead, most folks pull over at one of the dozens of convenient fast-food restaurants. Sometimes we are so busy with the details of daily living that we forget to appreciate the many pleasures and blessings that surround us. Pleasure becomes something that must be experienced quickly because there are other, more important issues to attend to. Why do we eat fast food instead of taking the time to prepare a good meal, for example? Life's little pleasures, such as preparing and enjoying a good meal, too often disappear from our busy days.

You love and appreciate food to the point that you'll try anything and wouldn't dare turn away a good brown butter sauce to go with your chicken. You'll order four desserts because each sounds so extraordinary. And you find the third glass of wine helps push any thought of healthy indulgence right out the window until tomorrow . . . and then tomorrow becomes a repeat of today. This tendency to say yes to every amazing food exacts a cost. Your body wears excess weight because the pleasure you find in eating overrides what you know is responsible and safe decision-making.

Remember, what goes in you sticks around to live on you. It's still possible to savor every meal and indulge your senses—just do so in moderation.

JUST 10 **STRATEGIES:** If you've gained weight because you're a sensual eater, I'd recommend that you rechannel some of your passion for food into other areas: reading, theater, crafts, music, walking, exercise, or even building friendships and strengthening relationships. And if you love to cook, you indulge this passion by getting creative with healthier versions of terrific recipes.

- **When you dine out, don't deny yourself a particular item.** Rather, watch portion sizes. Split an entrée or take half of it home with you. That way you can still enjoy everything.

- **Clear your palate, not your plate.** Once you've had your little taste, have a drink of water or brush your teeth. If the taste of that food lingers in your mouth, it will trigger more eating.

■ **Eat slowly.** It takes your brain at least 20 minutes to signal that your stomach is full. That may mean slowing down to take in the visual delights of a meal—something that should not be all that difficult for you as a food connoisseur.

YOUR AFFIRMATION: Today is a joyous day. I open my mind, heart, eyes, and ears to enjoy all the good things around me. I do not take them for granted. I enjoy my life, I enjoy my work, and I enjoy the people in my life. I trade terror for triumph, and frowns for smiles. I talk to myself in fun ways. I laugh. I use my good china. And if I want, I eat dessert first!

F. The Energy Eater

CHALLENGES: You do something most people do not: you listen to your hunger and feed it as necessary. But if you compensate for your hunger by eating more fast-acting carbohydrates—bread, crackers, granola bars—you could be consuming far more calories than you need while increasing your insulin production, which will, in turn, cause more hunger. I am this type of eater—even fit, trim, and healthy today.

You may also be easily overpowered by food cravings. It's long been thought that cravings arise from a nutritional deficit, but people crave salty foods, and few of us are salt-deficient.

So where else do these cravings come from?

Cravings for carbohydrates—sweets or starchy foods such as bread—can be triggered when your blood sugar is dipping low. This can be caused by going too long without eating or by filling up on sweets and caffeine.

Some research also suggests that cravings for sweets become worse when we don't eat enough complex carbohydrates. Carbohydrate cravings can also have an emotional basis, either as a rebellious response to an overly strict diet or as a learned choice for comfort.

Another popular theory is that cravings are hormonal. Changes in your hormonal levels can cause levels of the feel-good hormone serotonin to fluctuate. This can make you crave sweets and other carbs.

Another potential explanation for food cravings is a food allergy. Sometimes, the body's way of adapting to something that offends it is by craving it, much the same way that people crave nicotine or alcohol; if they stop eating the food to which they are allergic, they go through the same type of withdrawal. There are certain foods I largely avoid because I found that, once introduced, cravings would ensue without fail. So, I made them extinct! What foods fit this bill in your life?

JUST 10 **STRATEGIES:** If cravings strike only occasionally (on vacations or while traveling for work, for example) go ahead and eat a small portion without guilt. You're more likely to be satisfied with a small amount of the real thing. Cravings that strike more often may be helped by a change in eating habits. Also, you may want to travel with your favorite snacks and meal-replacement bars in your travel bag—I have a Shaklee's Cinch Bar with me at all times. When you are stuck and cannot sit down for a meal, grab a bar. Spread out your eating into three meals, with low-fat vegetable or fruit snacks as needed in between for hunger.

- **Watch your carbohydrates.** Look for fiber-rich, whole-grain cereals, breads, and crackers to fill a gap.

- **Schedule your treats.** Plan your daily menu, and include a couple of 100- to 150-calorie treats every now and then. Even if you think you'd never be able to eat chocolate again, you can eat it occasionally and still lose those 10 pounds.

- **Follow the 3-Hour Rule.** Stop eating three hours before bedtime and give yourself the gift of sleep by hitting the hay a half-hour earlier than normal. This will enable you to wake up ready for a good breakfast.

- **Walk for 15 minutes.** That's how long it took for a group of 25 chocoholics to exercise off their desire for a chocolate bar. This will get you moving and distracted from the need to eat. You'll forego the added calories, while burning calories on top of it.

■ **Take a whiff of mint.** A study at Wheeling Jesuit University in West Virginia found that people who sniffed peppermint periodically throughout the day ate 2,800 fewer calories during the week. When you focus on the scent, your attention is diverted away from cravings.

■ **Accept your cravings.** A study done at Drexel University found that people who had been taught to use techniques similar to mindful meditation were better able to resist a treat—in this case, a package of Hershey's Kisses—than those who didn't have the training. Mindfulness teaches that thoughts are just thoughts and don't require any rush to judgment or action. If you try to make them go away, all your focus is on the food. But if you just exist with the thought, it loses its power.

YOUR AFFIRMATION: I can eat whatever I want now, but I just don't need it. I know which foods are addictive to me, and I happily refuse them. When I make these choices, I give my thoughts and feelings instructions to move into a new state. I am patient but firm. I feel a new sense of freedom and peace. I am releasing my excess weight and its role, function, and purpose simultaneously. My whole outlook is changed; and I am grateful, happy, and optimistic.

Honor Your Body with Food

Many people with weight and food issues react to refined sugar, flour, and processed foods the way an alcoholic reacts to booze. One bite and sooner or later, there's a binge. To cleanse your system of foods that dishonor your body and lead to cravings, avoid these foods for at least 30 days. Give your body and mind time and space to detox.

When your body is not overloaded with too much junk food and fat, you have renewed energy. Your mind is sharper when it's not drugged by refined carbs. Your emotions are more serene and positive when you're not so full of self-hatred brought on by bad nutrition. Your body is no longer in an uproar. It is functioning calmly and efficiently. When you eat pure, wholesome foods, you feel better about yourself—and you feel better about your life.

The Love-Centered Food Plan helps you "get off" sugar and refined foods. It focuses on the following food groups.

Plant-Based Foods

"Eat your vegetables."

Remember how those three words struck horror in you as a kid? I bet you still remember sitting at the dinner table, hoping a dirty look could magically reduce that pile of peas or mountain of spinach.

Mom, and Grandma before her, didn't need surveys and scientific studies to know that the vitamins, minerals, and roughage provided by produce would help keep a body in proper working order.

But today those surveys and studies tell us even more. The most powerful argument for eating fruits and vegetables is their possible role as cancer fighters. Some studies found that people who eat few fruits and vegetables have about twice the risk of getting cancer as do people who eat lots of them.

The effects of increasing your consumption of fruits and vegetables can show up quickly on the scale. A Tufts University study found that the dieters who ate the widest variety of vegetables had the least amount of body fat. Vegetables are low in fat and calories, are a good source of dietary fiber, and provide us with extra energy. All these features help control weight effectively. You can consider fruits and vegetables your best friends in the Love-Centered Food Plan.

Life-Giving Protein

Protein is to your body what a wood frame is to your house or steel is to a bridge. Nutritionally, it is the most basic and important building material in your body, essential to high-level health because of its role in growth and maintenance. Your body breaks down protein from food into nutrient fragments called amino acids and reshuffles them into new protein to build and rebuild tissue, including body-firming muscle.

Protein also keeps your immune system functioning up to par, helps carry nutrients throughout the body, plays a part in forming hormones, and is involved in important enzyme reactions such as digestion.

It can also boost weight loss. In a study at the University of Illinois at Urbana-Champaign, women who exercised regularly and ate a reduced-calorie, high-protein diet lost more fat and less muscle than those who ate a similar diet high in carbohydrates.

Protein is thus indispensable to life because it plays a role in every part of the body and in every cell.

Healthy Fats

Fat is not a bad word or the source of all dietary evil. In fact, fat is one of three macronutrients that human beings need to survive. (The other two are protein and carbohydrates.) Generally speaking, the most healthful fats are found in some—but not all—vegetable oils. They have no cholesterol, provide essential fatty acids, and are—with a few exceptions—highly unsaturated. (Saturated fats, on the other hand, are linked to heart disease and other serious illnesses.)

When you eat from the Love-Centered Food Plan, you'll choose healthy fats, mostly vegetable oils and omega-3 fatty acids from fish. Omega-3s may promote weight loss by helping stabilize blood sugar and boosting mood (depression can lead to overeating and vice versa).

The Love-Centered Diet offers a wonderful way for you to start loving your body. And when you love your body, it will love you back!

The Love-Centered Food Plan

This plan is not your next new diet, nor the latest fad. It's based on making simple, healthy food choices that will help you lose weight right now. I wouldn't say it's easy, but it's simple. Here's what you eat.

PROTEINS		
3¼ Servings Daily		
Beef, lean cuts	Fish	Shellfish, including clams, crab, lobster, oysters, scallops, and shrimp
Cheese	Lamb	Soy protein
Chicken breast	Milk (low-fat) and low-fat buttermilk	Turkey
Cottage cheese (low-fat)	Pork, lean cuts	Turkey bacon
Eggs	Sausage, lean	Yogurt (low-fat)
FIBROUS VEGETABLES		
Specified in the 30-day meal plan		
Asparagus	Garlic	Radishes
Broccoli	Greens (all types: beet, collard, mustard, spinach, turnip, etc.)	Sauerkraut
Brussels sprouts	Green beans	Sprouts, all varieties
Cabbage	Leeks	Summer squash
Cauliflower	Lettuce, all varieties	Tomatoes
Celery	Onions	Yellow (wax) beans
Chard	Parsley	Zucchini
Cucumbers	Peppers, all varieties, hot and sweet	
Eggplant	Pickles	
STARCHY VEGETABLES		
1–2 Servings Daily		
Beets	Peas	Turnips
Carrots	Pumpkin	Winter squashes
Parsnips	Sweet potatoes	

FRUITS		
2–3 Servings Daily		
Apples, all varieties	Honeydew melon	Peaches
Apricots	Kiwi	Pears
Berries, all varieties	Lemons	Plums
Cantaloupe	Limes	Tangerines
Casaba melon	Nectarines	Watermelon
Grapefruit	Oranges	
HEALTHY OILS AND FATS		
Up to 3 Servings Daily (small amounts of oil or oil spray to cook protein do not count toward your daily total)		
Butter	Olive oil, extra-virgin	Soybean oil
Canola oil	Salad dressings, (low sugar)	Sunflower oil
Grapeseed oil	Sesame oil	Walnut oil

In the next section you will find a "blueprint" to show you how the Love-Centered Diet is structured. It will help you with your own meal planning.

The Love-Centered Diet Blueprint

BREAKFAST
1¼ protein
1 fruit
Example: 2 large scrambled or poached eggs, 1 cup fresh berries, and ¼ cup plain yogurt

LUNCH
1 protein
2 fibrous vegetables
1 fat
1 fruit
Example: One 4-ounce chicken breast (skinless, baked or grilled), 1 cup of steamed green beans, 1 cup of garden salad with up to 1 tablespoon oil or dressing, and 1 cup berries

DINNER
1 protein
1 starchy vegetable
1 fibrous vegetable
2 fats
Example: One 4-ounce salmon fillet (broiled or baked), 1 cup steamed peas, large mixed green salad (approximately 1½ cups raw salad veggies), and 2 tablespoons oil or salad dressing

SNACKS
1 fruit serving
Example: 1 medium apple

BEVERAGES
Water, sparkling water, or flavored water
Coffee or tea

Mastering Portion Control

People who successfully maintain their weight over the long term do not go hog wild and eat everything in sight. Quite the contrary. They practice portion control, and you must do the same. If you eat what you've been eating, you'll weigh what you've weighed, so get on board with me here and focus on the first 10 pounds. Hunger pangs will not hurt you and, in fact, are a brilliant sign that your body is coming to life and getting out of the numb, stuffed state it's been in for so long. So, portion control!

If you've had lap band or gastric bypass surgery, which physically makes three meals a day impossible, split your meals up to five instead of three (same amounts, just over two extra smaller meals) and follow your physician's guidance on spacing. Other than these two exceptions, it's three meals and a snack and the "how much?" matters a lot. It's portion control, portion control, portion control.

Your Love-Centered Food Plan requires that you continue to eat specific quantities of food. Be aware of what constitutes a serving, and don't fudge it by taking more than what is allotted. You'll find that your food plan has more than enough food to satisfy your hunger and feed your body. Serving sizes are listed in the chart below.

Food Group	Serving Size
Proteins	4 ounces cooked lean meat, poultry, or fish (about the size of a deck of cards or the palm of your hand)
	Other foods that count as protein: 2 eggs; 3 slices of turkey bacon; 2 ounces of cheese (the size of a domino); and 1 cup skim milk, low-fat milk, soy milk, cottage cheese, or yogurt
Fibrous Vegetables	Portions set in the 30-day meal plan
Starchy Vegetables	½ cup steamed beets, pumpkin, sweet potato, or winter squash; or 1cup steamed carrots, parsnips, peas, or turnips
Fruits	1 medium piece of raw fruit; ½ grapefruit; ½ melon; 1 cup berries; 3 small fruits (apricots, tangerines, kiwis, lemons, or limes), 1 apple
Fats	1 tablespoon of oil, salad dressing, or butter

Eat Seasonally

When shopping, learn to eat seasonally for freshness and good value. For example, look for asparagus, leaf lettuce, spinach, and peas in the spring; strawberries, blueberries, peaches, peppers, tomatoes, and broccoli in the summer; and apples, pears, squash, and sweet potatoes in the fall.

There are a number of good reasons to eat seasonally. It helps to support the local and regional economy; but even more vital, seasonal food is fresher and therefore tends to be tastier and more nutritious.

The recipes in this book are organized seasonally, although feel free to prepare them at any time of the year.

Spices and Condiments

Get creative with spices, herbs, and low-sugar condiments such as low-sodium soy sauce, Tabasco, Worcestershire sauce, tomato sauce and paste, and onion soup mix. Make sure not to eat too much sodium. Most of the sodium Americans ingest is in processed foods. When you're on the *Just 10* diet, you can add a little salt to flavor without going nuts. I love a little Mrs. Dash, the no-salt seasonings in a bottle.

My Five Alive Rule

If buying processed food products is unavoidable, be sure to read the nutrition labels. Make sure sugar is the fifth (or later) item on the ingredient list—the further down the list the better. If sugar (in any form—sucrose, fructose, and so on) is the first, second, third, or fourth ingredient, then skip it! The only exception I make is when I'm on the road and using meal replacement options, but keep in mind, certain brands are better than others. I like Shaklee's Cinch shakes and bars because they are high in protein, low in calories, and gluten free. Crunched for time? Have what I call your "emergency food" on hand like a Cinch Bar—don't skip a meal, no matter what. Make sure to use low-glycemic sweeteners as this indicates a slower rate of digestion and therefore a slower blood-sugar absorption rate. I prefer brown rice syrup or honey over white sugar any day. Avoiding high fructose corn syrup altogether is a good idea, since it is such a pervasive ingredient in the typical American diet.

And what about artificial sweeteners? Go easy on these—no more than three packets daily. (This was a biggie for me, as I weaned myself from 20 servings of the yellow-packeted sweetener a day in food and drinks, to just 2 pink packets.) Be sure to keep an eye out because these sweeteners seem to be everywhere—in diet and even nondiet drinks, many foods and snack bars, and even many of the candy, breath mints, and gum you've come to depend on. I want you to move toward removing these fake foods, these FrankenFoods, altogether.

Reclaim Your (Food) Chain

FrankenFood is engineered to make you taste something in a certain way, other than how nature intended. The result on the human brain is often this response: MORE! As in, feed me more, give me more, "I WANT MORE!"

We're inundated with genetically modified food (GMF) made from genetically modified organisms (GMO). Falling into *Just 10* with me involves reclaiming your food chain by getting rid of the junk food so many are hooked on.

These include the biggies like fake sweeteners, high fructose corn syrup, refined grains, and FrankenFood sweeteners, but there are thousands more.

There's a movement in this country to make food manufacturers label foods that have been genetically altered, and if you ask me, it's about time. While some genetically modified foods have benefits, most are designed to extend shelf-life stability and to make you, the consumer, crave more of it.

GMFs are generally less nutritious than real food, and they make us eat more than we should. As a result, GMFs contribute significantly to obesity.

Consider just one little itsy bitsy artificial sweetener—Aspartame, or NutraSweet. Are you aware it's in over 6,000 products? And do you know the possible health effects of consuming this and other artificial sweet stuff?

See the chart below for all the nasty things various sweeteners can do to our bodies. Manufacturers are sneaking FrankenFood sweeteners into energy bars, drinks, syrups, cakes, gum, and candies because it's so much cheaper to use than real sugar. Be alert—if it's not natural, it's not a way to take good care of yourself, and it's best to stay away from it.

COMMON SWEETENERS ADDED TO FOODS		
Sweetener	Food Sources	Potential Ill Effects
Acesulfame-K	Sugar-free baked goods, chewing gum, gelatin desserts, and soft drinks	Possible carcinogen

Aspartame (the blue packet)	Diet products and sugar substitutes (such as NutraSweet), including soft drinks, drink mixes, gelatin desserts, and low-calorie frozen desserts	Possible increased cancer risk with lifelong use
Corn syrup	Candy, marshmallows, syrups, snack foods, and imitation dairy foods	No nutritional value other than calories, promotes tooth decay
Dextrose	Bread, caramel candies, soda pop, cookies, and many other foods	No nutritional value other than calories, promotes tooth decay
Sweetener	**Food Sources**	**Potential Ill Effects**
Fructose	"Health" drinks and other products	Increases triglyceride (fat) levels and risk of heart disease, affects appetite-regulating hormones, and contributes to weight gain
High fructose corn syrup (HFCS)	Soft drinks, juices, other processed foods	Implicated in obesity, heart disease, and possibly cancer
Rebiana	Diet products and sugar substitutes (such as Truvia)	Unknown to date
Saccharin (the pink packet)	Diet products and sugar substitutes (such as Sweet'N Low)	Possible carcinogen. I believe it's the safest of artificial sweeteners.
Sucralose (the yellow packet)	Diet products, sugar substitutes (such as Splenda), no-added-sugar baked goods, frozen desserts, ice cream, and soft drinks	Inconclusive, implicated in cancer and immune system problems
Sugar (sucrose)	Table sugar, sweetened foods	Promotes tooth decay, promotes obesity and heart disease in people with high triglycerides
Sugar alcohols	Candy, chocolates, baked goods, ice cream, and also diet products	Poorly absorbed in the body, can cause diarrhea

Adapted from various research studies.

Based on the foods and serving sizes listed above, I've developed a sample 30-day food plan with recipes. You will find this at the end of the book in the section titled *"Just 10*—The 30-Day Plan." Follow it as closely as you can—and watch the pounds melt off.

Take 10

1. Eat breakfast! People who skip this critical meal end up eating more calories throughout the day.

2. Is a tall glass of juice your morning ritual? Swap that glass of OJ for a real orange and you not only save more than 50 calories, you also get some fiber while you're at it. Fruit juices are a low-fiber, high-calorie staple you can stand to lose.

3. Choose darker salad greens such as red leaf and green leaf lettuces, which have more nutrients than lighter greens such as iceberg. Spinach and mâche are terrific choices, too, and they are available at your local farmers' market and most grocery stores.

4. Remove the skin from a chicken breast after cooking and save 100 calories each time.

5. Eat all your meals! In our busy lives, skipping meals is a constant temptation. If you are on the go and cannot get the meal you'd planned, then substitute with a meal-replacement bar or shake.

6. Broil, bake, braise, steam, stir-fry, poach, grill, sauté (with minimal oils), boil, and roast on racks. There are so many ways to cook your meals, and they start with how you take the food from raw to cooked. All these are self-loving solutions to the instinct to fry.

7. Eat slowly. Take at least 20 minutes for meals and 10 minutes for snacks so that you'll feel more satisfied with

smaller food quantities and will therefore eat less than those who eat fast. It takes 20 minutes for the brain to receive the signal from the stomach saying, "I'm full."

8. Choose one specific location to eat and make eating a singular activity. Beware of unconscious eating—in front of the TV; at the movies; or while reading, studying, driving, cooking, or standing. When you're involved in an activity while eating, you can be distracted from really tasting or enjoying your food, which makes it easy to overeat.

9. Jazz up plain water with juice from a quarter of a lemon or other fruit. It's simple but good.

10. Control emotional eating. Don't reach for food to make you feel content or more relaxed. Food is not the answer.

JUST 10 MYTH BUSTER
I CAN'T CHANGE

We've all heard the expressions "A leopard can't change his spots" and "You can't teach an old dog new tricks." Both imply that we can't change our established patterns of opinion and behavior, because these are our "nature."

I disagree. Think of how often you've heard someone say, "This book changed my life," or "I didn't know any better at that age, but I see things differently now."

Examine your own life. How much of your life is the same as when you were 15, 25, or 35? If you have deliberately tried to keep things the same, how successful would you have been? Have you grown, developed, or matured in significant ways?

My guess is that your answer was yes. So, the bottom line is that neither our personalities nor our behavior is perpetually fixed. Each of us can change.

Technically, a leopard's spots can't change, but the leopard can climb a different tree now and then. As for dogs, it's quite possible to teach an old dog—or in this case, a human—new "tricks," or new behaviors.

We rescued our dog Harriet, and she had more than a bag of behavioral issues. Truth be told, at times even I was afraid of her. She growled. She lunged at people. She bared her teeth more often than I wish to remember. We wondered what we might do—could we really teach her to be unafraid, to stay connected, and to trust? We used love and consistency as the approach and eventually it worked. Over time, and with work, Harriet became less afraid; more trusting; and a happier, healthier part of the family.

Consider these inspiring examples, too: George Burns received his first Academy Award when he was 80. At 71, Golda Meir became prime minister of Israel. And Julia Child began cooking in her 40s and got her own television show when she was 50.

So remember this: Lots of "old dogs" become award-winning artists, start businesses, run countries, and learn all sorts of new skills and behaviors. We can all learn how to sit, stay, roll over—and change!

CHAPTER TWO

STEP
2

Start a Moving Meditation

M ost of us don't like to exercise. We'd rather spend extra time looking for a parking space that is right next to the store than walk a few minutes through a parking lot. We'll go out of our way *not* to move. It's too bad, really.

To optimize weight loss and gain overall fitness, we need to move, some way, somehow. Our bodies were designed for what I call "loving movement," in combination with a diet of healthy food

There are so many exciting new findings about exercise. For instance, a Harvard Alumni Study of 16,000 people found a direct relationship between the number of exercise calories burned per week and overall longevity. The more calories participants expended in physical activity, the longer they lived. Not a bad investment if you ask me!

Even cooler: exercise makes brain cells more energetic. They grow, branch out, and make connections to one another. In a 2006 study by University of Illinois researchers, 30 healthy but sedentary men and women ages 60 to 79 were put on an aerobic exercise training program. After six months, their brain volume—the amount of gray and white matter—had increased. That meant more brain cells and more connections between them. (Brain volume didn't increase in 30 similar people who participated in a toning and stretching program.) The researchers explained that aerobic exercise increases the supply of a protein called brain-derived neurotrophic factor (BDNF), which protects brain cells and promotes the growth of new nerve cells and synapses that are related to learning and memory. For me, this means I can reverse the damage I did to my brain as a result of all my years of drinking, smoking, and drugging.

Exercise also acts as a great antidepressant. In a study published in the September 2007 issue of *Psychosomatic Medicine*, researchers observed 202 men and women age 40 and older with major depression. They randomly assigned the participants to one of four groups: one that exercised in a supervised group setting three times per week, one that exercised alone at home three times per week, one that took the antidepressant sertraline, and one that took a placebo. Those in the exercise groups worked out for the same amount of time whether they were working out in groups or alone at home. They began with a 10-minute warm-up, followed by 30 minutes of walking or jogging on a treadmill, and then finished with a 5-minute cool-down.

By the end of the 16-week study, nearly half of the people in the exercise groups no longer met the criteria for major depression. This is the same rate of success as the group taking the sertraline, showing that regular exercise is as effective as this prescription antidepressant. All treatments were more effective than the placebo.

So why do so many people still resist getting off their proverbial butt? Probably because exercise feels too much like homework, something we have to do.

I have a new solution. It's time to forget that exercise is about pushing yourself to do a particular workout—like running for 30 minutes or going to a spinning class three times a week—or forcing yourself to exercise at dawn when you're not a morning person. Exercise shouldn't add stress to your life. Gone are the days of saying, "I must exercise!"

Instead, think about exercise as a "moving meditation," which may sound more appealing. When you move—without being pressured or guilted into it, without dreading it—the pounds come off effortlessly as long as you do it several times a week. Moving meditation is walking, jogging, running, swimming, or biking while focusing only on your breathing, your body in motion, the scenery around you, or the spiritual force in your life. Take off the head-phones and move, breathe, and just be.

Let me elaborate on this definition by telling you a story. Years ago, I decided to learn meditation to take advantage of its well-known benefits. Most of the forms of meditation I was familiar with focused on sitting and breathing without thought for a specific amount of time. In my ignorance, I thought it sounded pretty simple. After all, I managed to pass several college classes using that technique.

In an effort to focus my mind and be fully present, I tried medi-tating on candle flames, mantras, and my navel but to no avail. At that point, I happily threw in the meditation towel and headed to the woods for a nice, long walk. That's where I would eventually discover the power of "moving meditation."

The wind stirring a tree's leaves began to sound like beauti-ful music. I loved lingering near a fragrant flower, leaning in for a moment to inhale. Walking on a recently trod horse trail taught me to be visually aware of my surroundings, too. As I immersed myself in nature on a regular basis, I learned to be in the moment. The now, the here, became dear and noticed. A thought jumped out at me: in that moment, when I was focused on myself, my breath, and my spirit moving freely and celebrating life, I got an enormous dose of love from the universe. It was like a big beautiful karma-boomerang of love. Small world, big love.

The new habits of nurturing myself and having powerful con-versations with my own spirit sprang from all of this. I didn't realize I was doing moving meditation until I had been doing it for years.

How to Do a Moving Meditation

A moving meditation can involve any form of activity, from yoga to swimming to biking, as long as you consciously pay attention to experiencing the present moment. Even on a stationary bike, just taking the time out to be alone with yourself, to stop and collect your thoughts, can be meditative. That's why I encourage people to exercise mindfully, so they're present in their bodies instead of just thinking about dinner or checking their minds at the door.

Exercise can provide a wonderful reflective space if done mindfully. Your moving meditation helps connect your body with the mind and spirit. The results can range from reduced stress to communion with the divine. Here are some examples of moving meditations you may want to try.

Walking

A walking meditation is the easiest. You can do it anywhere—walking to your car, around the mall, in your neighborhood, or on a walking track. Turn off your electronic devices and disconnect from your busy, hectic life.

To do a walking meditation:

1. Begin walking at your usual pace, relaxing your body as you move. (Good walking shoes are important, too.)

2. Coordinate your breath to your walk. For instance, you might take three steps for each inhalation and three for each exhalation. Keep a steady pace, using your breath as a guide.

3. As you walk, notice how your feet hit the ground. Continue for 5 to 10 minutes. Eventually you'll be able to do this for 20 minutes or more.

When I do my walking meditation, I feel that I am part of something larger—the road beneath me, the trees that shade parts of my walk, the green spikes of grass at the side of the street. I'm removed from the physicality of my movements, in sync with the steady beat of my feet hitting the pavement. I actually feel more energized and focused at the end of this kind of walk than after a power walk designed to burn calories.

The emphasis is always to make walking a joyful, healthy, lifelong activity, because it is a "practice" instead of exercise. You can literally do this anywhere, anytime. I always encourage walkers to exercise outdoors and preferably in nature . . . off the paved path. That's where the deeper enjoyment lies!

By transforming walking into a mindful practice, you'll discover so many benefits on all levels: physical, mental, emotional, and even spiritual, because it lets you experience a deeper sense of inner peace. And this goes way beyond the endorphin-induced "runner's high" we always hear about.

Dance

I recommend dancing as a moving meditation. Not only does it feel good and offer a great workout (without you realizing it!) but it can also tap into a primal part of you. The rhythms of the music and the movement of your body evoke your spirit and soul. And dancing doesn't require any special skill, only a desire to try. We can enjoy dancing throughout our entire lives. There are so many forms— ballroom, ballet, Latin, belly dancing, swing, Zumba, and so forth.

Dance gives you as much strength, suppleness, tone, and balance as "straightforward" exercise. And because you dance to music in a social setting, you're in a better frame of mind to work out. I think it's one of the best ways to express yourself, relieve stress, and stay in shape.

Classes are abundant in most cities, so you shouldn't have much trouble finding one that's right for you. Look online, or you can try contacting a fitness center, community college, community recreation program, dance studio, or dance club in your area.

Yoga

Yoga is a wonderful form of moving meditation that is accepted worldwide. This wasn't always the case. As a boy growing up in Eugene, Oregon, I went to school one morning and found my third-grade teacher had gone away for a week. In her place was a guitar-playing, granola-eating, meditating, yoga-practicing substitute teacher by the name of Sunny. I found her fascinating.

Excited, I raced home from school and told my parents all about my new teacher. Being strict evangelical Quakers, they were horrified; and in short order, they called the school. Soon, McCormick Elementary School gave the boot to this lovely "Eastern-religion-pushing" sub.

That was 1973, when most people associated yoga with free love, flower power, and limber old gurus in white robes wrapping their heels behind their ears. Today everyone is doing it, from housewives and pop stars to athletes and school kids. It's obvious to me how much yoga has grown in popularity.

Yoga's big attraction is that it works wonders. Research, much of it done in India, suggests a wide variety of positive health benefits—for arthritis, asthma, heart disease, and some cancers, among other things. Many yogalike postures, stretches, and positions are used today by athletes, rehab programs, and physical therapists. A lot of people who take up yoga find that it may actually cure their lower back pain.

To do yoga right, you really have to focus your attention inward and quiet your mind. Yoga encourages long, deep breaths that slow your heart rate, lower your blood pressure, and ease anxiety. The whole activity—the stretching, balancing, breathing—makes the stress and strain of the day melt away and really helps you center yourself emotionally and spiritually.

Modern yoga is exercise, not a religion; and the yoga we do now isn't really thousands of years old, either. There are so many different forms. The word *yoga* means "to join," to bring together the mind and body. Breathing is used as a way to focus and link the mind to the way the body works.

In a culture that worships youth, yoga honors the aging process. Poses can be modified to every body type and level of ability, making yoga accessible to anyone willing to step onto the mat. And the philosophy of the practice encourages accepting what is happening in the present moment.

Yoga is taught everywhere in the United States—in gyms, at YMCAs, on television and DVDs, and in private yoga studios. Good instructors will show you how to progress at your own pace. A yoga class or session goes by quickly, too, because you're switching constantly from one position to another. You're also holding positions, and this builds strength. Yoga offers both variety and an athletic challenge. Plus, it's perfect for people of all ages. And don't worry about whether or not you're flexible enough to try the positions in the first place. Maybe you can't bend backward far enough so that your head brushes the floor, but everybody has sufficient flexibility to do some yoga.

Tai Chi

Most of you reading this step have already formed a mental picture of how tai chi works. It's that slow-moving person doing those dancelike movements in the park early in the morning, right? That's right, but tai chi is much more than that. It is a style of martial arts that has tremendous health benefits.

Tai chi focuses on stimulating a person's "chi," or life force. Chi is in and around us, and we want it to do the work for us, instead of relying solely on our muscles. If we set up the body correctly by relaxing and aligning it, we can become a conduit for the flow of chi. Chi goes into the deepest parts of our bodies, including bone marrow, to energize health and healing.

The actual moves involve shifting the body's weight from leg to leg with slow deliberate movements, while the arms and hands sweep in front and beside the body. Each position in tai chi requires concentration and a certain amount of control to perform correctly.

I like tai chi for its variety and many benefits. It has aspects of martial arts, but it is also a form of low-impact exercise that is definitely a moving meditation.

No-Weight Workout

I love it when people want to do some strength training (also called weight training). It makes visible changes to your shape. It helps your metabolism. And it improves your body image and self-esteem. Seeing your muscles reveal themselves after only a few short weeks is so empowering.

Science backs me up on this. Several years ago, researchers in North Carolina discovered that getting college women on a strength-training program made them love and appreciate their bodies. In fact, many of the women who were classified as "body-image disturbed" prior to the study changed their attitudes so much that they could no longer be put in this classification. The researchers concluded, "These results provide evidence to suggest that weight training may be an effective treatment for body image disturbance."

But can strength training be a moving meditation? Yes! As you do strength-training exercises, allow your mind to enter a meditative zone. Shut out distractions around you. Focus on the muscle you're working. Draw your attention inward so that you become aware of your body getting stronger under your skin. Tap into your inner energy and feel it circulating as you move. Any exercise can be meditative.

I recommend a basic strength-training program to my weight-coaching clients. I call it the "No-Weight Workout." It provides a simple, accessible way to move without picking up weights, dropping dumbbells, or going to a gym. You'll find my No-Weight Workout in Appendix A.

What I hope to have gotten across in this chapter is that moving meditations can be fun and good for your soul. They can open you up in many ways. Don't be afraid to try something new. Venturing into a yoga class or a dance class takes courage, but it could change your life. And if classes are too much for you right now, simply dance in front of a mirror to drink in your beautiful body as it is, because it soon will change. Turn on your favorite music and dance with your eyes closed, listening to your breath as you move and shake and bend and celebrate your body. Or do yoga to a DVD in the comfort of your own home. Check out our No-Weight Workout and *Just 10* yoga sessions with my buddy Bryant Stiney at *Just10Diet.com*. It won't cost you a dime, and I know you'll find it helpful and inspiring.

Soon you will see that moving meditation makes you feel better, and you will want to continue. So adopt this as your new exercise paradigm. Your body will gravitate toward a healthy, comfortable weight for you. Along the way, you'll achieve a peaceful, positive way of looking at your life and loving yourself.

Take 10

1. Select a moving meditation that will be fun for you. Find one that allows you to get in touch with your inner self, meet new people, or learn new skills. And make sure you would do it for a lifetime. You really have to enjoy it that much.

2. Make time. Learn how to add just 10 minutes of a moving meditation a day. The goal is 30 minutes a day. If you walk for just 30 minutes—even just three 10-minute walks a day—you can lose 10 extra pounds this year.

3. Do your moving meditation at your favorite time of day. If yours is an outdoor moving meditation, practice it in scenery that uplifts you. Choose whatever environment makes you feel comfortable, wear whatever you like, but use the workout to get in touch with your body and clear your mind.

4. Define and set goals in your journal or *Just 10 Workbook*. Your goals do not always have to be lofty, hard-to-attain ones. Set smaller, attainable goals, such as doing your moving meditation at least three times a week for 30 minutes each time. Each week, increase your goal incrementally. Every goal you achieve builds momentum toward the next.

5. Keep your focus on your very own *Just 10 Lbs.* goal. It's doable! Attainable! Enjoy the activity; and do it for fun, meditation, and spiritual connection.

6. Write down your activities in your journal or *Just 10 Workbook*. Note how you feel after each "work-in," including your energy levels and mood. Write about the accomplishment of being joyously active.

7. Put some variety into your moving meditation. Do different activities during the week. Skip the walk one day, and try a dance or yoga class. Experiment!

8. Don't look back. Don't dwell on your years of overeating and other bad habits. Be proud of your accomplishments today. Meditate on those as you move.

9. If the words "I don't feel like exercising today" enter your mind, it's time to reboot your thinking. Remind yourself that "feeling like it" isn't a prerequisite for sticking to your plan. Think of it this way: you don't always feel like going to work, calling your parents, or mowing the lawn, but you do these things anyway because they're necessary.

10. Make your moving meditation a priority. After establishing momentum, you'll be more inclined to eat healthfully. The involvement, the feeling of accomplishment, however small, will give you the boost you need to keep going.

JUST 10 MYTH BUSTER
EXERCISE MUST BE STRENUOUS
TO BE BENEFICIAL

Your body was designed to move, so any type of activity is good for you. It's not necessary to push yourself to extremes to get the benefits, either. Always think "moving meditation" rather than exercise. Dancing, yoga, gardening, and nature walks are all beneficial forms of movement. And they may actually be safer than more strenuous forms of exercise. In addition to the risk of injury, overexerting yourself can suppress immunity and put your heart at risk. Before starting any new exercise program, see your physician for a checkup to make sure you don't check out.

CHAPTER THREE

STEP 3 Develop a Daily Practice

ecause you're reading this book and working your way through each of its steps, I know that you clearly *intend* to lose 10 pounds. Step 3 will solidify that intention so it becomes real. This step creates success by helping you determine exactly what your life will look like, day by day. And each healthy, successful day gets you closer to a thinner, fitter body.

I'm not a mind reader, but I'm pretty sure I know what success looks like for you:

Experiencing life as a thin, healthy person...no longer having a huge weight literally holding you back from truly living, jumping, running, and playing...participating in fun sports and activities, not just being a spectator...shopping at normal stores, not just those that carry plus-size clothes...no longer worrying about fitting into seats in airplanes, theaters, restaurants, and amusement parks...not fearing a future of diabetes, heart attacks, strokes, sleep apnea, or other weight-related health issues...experiencing sexual connectedness without fear or body shame...being in control of your appetites and habits instead of being controlled by them. (By the way, if you haven't set your desires on these things, it's time to get in intention mode!)

Create Value-Aligned Intentions

Your reasons for wanting to be thin must be aligned with things you value, or even the best intentions to lose weight will fail. In other words, they must be "value aligned." To make that happen, add at least one mindful, compelling reason—that is, a motivator—to your intention. This is like creating a vision statement of who or where you want to be in the future.

Case in point: "I will lose 10 pounds (intention), so I can get my energy back, which means I can participate in activities with friends and family—(motivator)." When you're clear about your values, you're drawn toward what you want, and you'll react strongly against anything that pulls you away from it.

When you live according to value-aligned intentions, your focus automatically narrows considerably. Consciously choosing to be thin and healthy shifts your energy from unwise actions and draws you toward positive ones. You make the choices and take the actions to get there. The clearer your value-aligned intention, the more power you have. But you have to set that intention each day—that is what a daily practice is all about.

The Power of a Daily Practice

Every day that you work toward losing the next pound, there will be challenges. Cravings arise. Barriers surface. Frustrations mount. Temptations leap out of nowhere. But if we take special time, daily, to prepare our hearts, minds, and responses—everything that squares with our value-aligned intention—no problem or challenge is too much for us to handle.

And so, to get the next pound off, you must start each day with a daily practice, a collection of conscious, peaceful actions that sets the pace for your entire day. It could involve doing 10 minutes of yoga, sipping herbal tea in your garden, or having moments of quiet reflection. Daily practice is a form of meditation, but it entails a specific commitment you make to yourself, a ritual you perform each morning as a way of honoring your value-aligned intention.

There is nothing new about a daily practice. In ancient rituals, people rose in the morning and turned toward the sun, honoring the source of light and warmth that sustained all life. Even on cloudy days they turned in the sun's direction and honored the source they knew to be present. All major faiths have morning rituals, from prayers to special readings. The purpose is to give special meaning to your life and set a positive course for the day.

Here's why a daily practice is critical to your success: When you awaken each morning, you face a new beginning. It doesn't matter what happened or didn't happen yesterday. Whatever it was, it was yesterday, it is gone, finished, no longer a part of your life. Forget it, release it, and let it go.

The beginning, which is right now, is the time to set your intentions for the day—to eat healthy, to move your body, and to let go of the old thoughts in your mind. You can eagerly look forward each day to new interests and new joys and feel like a new creature, strong, free, radiant, and whole.

The benefits of a daily practice begin when you start the activity. They include reducing anxiety, increasing your focus on priorities in the day and in your life, and building an internal serenity that guides you. But the benefits extend far beyond the mere minutes you spend on your practice.

I often refer to daily practice as "meditative relaxation" because your body is calm while your mind is engaged. In a state of meditative relaxation, your heart rate slows, blood pressure normalizes, and breathing quiets. The echo of your daily practice will resonate throughout your day. Studies have shown that the longer people do a daily practice like this, the younger they score on tests of biological age. Now that's real rejuvenation!

All of these benefits keep you moving in the direction of your goal: a fit, healthy body. The important part of this is that you do it every day—so that you get to know your body, awaken your mind, and connect with your spirit.

How to Establish Your Daily Practice

Establishing a personal daily practice requires some commitment and a change to your routine—but no special skill. If you are able to sit comfortably with your eyes closed, in a relatively quiet environment, you can do it.

My own daily practice is to roll out of bed and do 15 minutes of meditation, sit-ups, push-ups, and stretching. I even glide my hands over my body to connect with my own body image. I never skip my daily practice, because I love what it does for me. It keeps me focused on what I want in life, and it's essential for maintaining a healthy lifestyle.

A daily practice is different for each person. However, let me give you some important guidelines on how to get started.

Create Sacred Spaces within Your Home

I believe a productive daily practice must take place in a peaceful environment, free from clutter and distraction. Clearing away clutter in your home allows you to clear away the mental mess.

I admit that it can be hard to keep all of the rooms of your home clean and tidy all of the time. I realize things can get a little chaotic, between junk mail, the kids' muddy soccer cleats, the home office, and pet toys. An easy way to figure out what to declutter is to do a quick inventory of your house. Walk around your home with a sheet of paper and catalog messy areas or places where the energy feels chaotic. After you've made your list, choose the top areas that feel like they could use the most attention, and declutter those. Reduce the amount of "stuff" you have and you'll feel liberated.

With some conscious choices and clear boundaries, you can create pockets in your home that feel like sacred spaces. For example, if you like to meditate, create a meditation room or even just a meditation corner. Include special pillows, a prayer shawl, candles, a cross, and spiritual icons—anything that supports you. This area can be your sacred space, where you can do your daily practice. For instance, in my home, I like the wood floor in the second-floor bedroom near the windows. A tranquil place all by itself. And it is a great location for my daily practice.

As you prepare for your daily practice, make sure to cut out distractions. Turn your phone ringers off. Turn on a radio station or a CD of soothing sounds such as the ocean, or a babbling brook, or a fireplace crackling. If you wish, set the atmosphere with dimmed lights, scented candlelight, or no lights at all.

Focus on Your Intentions

During your daily practice, I'd like you to focus on thoughts and visions of fulfilling your *Just 10* weight goal. There are several ways to do this. Let me share them with you now.

Visualization

When you visualize, you see in your mind's eye the body that you would like to have and/or the life you would like to be living at your new healthy weight. Visualize the perfectly healthy day you're going to have *today*. This technique is very powerful and many successful people—from elite athletes to top businesspeople—use it to achieve their goals.

Visualization is very simple. Settle in to your sacred space or some other comfortable place. Make sure that you won't be disturbed.

Now try to imagine yourself the way you would like to be. Visualize your body as you would like it to look. What is your weight? What is your waist like? What do your legs look like?

See yourself in motion, such as in a film . . . walking on the beach . . . playing a sport . . . entering a room in a flattering dress. Try to get a clear image in your mind. Maintain the image long enough that the mental picture you create evokes an emotional response. The emotion causes conviction, and conviction causes reality.

Visualization has a huge impact on your subconscious mind. Your subconscious mind does not distinguish between whether you're imagining something or actually experiencing it. It thus makes your brain want to work toward your goal. When that happens, you will achieve it. You're giving instructions to your subconscious mind to move into this new state. This is very powerful stuff.

Breathing is important, too. As you breathe, inhale your vision or intention, then exhale those things that no longer serve you—such as out-of-control eating or sedentary habits.

You can also take this technique further and think of what you need to do to fulfill your intention. This is important. Spend time visualizing the day ahead. See yourself eating only healthy food and doing your moving meditation during the day. Visualize yourself becoming more fit each day. This technique is not only applicable to weight loss, it can be used for anything you want in life.

Chanting

Chanting can be singing or speaking, simply saying a word or phrase over and over again to calm, focus, and let go. Settle in to your sacred place and simply begin speaking or singing. Go with anything, just to get started and release tension. When I first tried this style of relaxation, I said again and again, "My God loves me, and I am safe in this moment."

As you begin, start by repeating a phrase or a short affirmation that helps you set your value-aligned intention. Some examples of short affirmations:

- Today, I manifest health, strength, and bodily renewal.

- I am vitally alive.

- I am filled with energy.

- I am radiant with good health.

- I am happy and enthusiastic about life and living.

- I make good choices today. I choose health.

- Today, I choose to react calmly and creatively to challenges that confront me.

- I am calm and relaxed around all food.

Say it quietly or loudly, depending on how you're feeling.

Repeat the phrase for two minutes every day for two to three days, then extend the duration of your practice. If you find yourself distracted by visual stimulation, close your eyes. Before you know it, you're chanting. Don't be afraid. It's a rich way to self-soothe and cultivate calmness.

Prayer

Prayer is a conversation with God. It has probably been practiced since the dawn of humanity and is an essential ingredient in the world's major religions. It is the primary activity of most private devotions.

Most Christian prayers end with *amen*, Hebrew for "so be it," which makes it a very powerful, affirming word. Muslims are required to repeat short prayers in Arabic five times each day as they face Mecca. Buddhists often employ prayer as a meditative tool, while Hindus vigorously chant the names of God, sing the praises of deities, and participate in elaborate ritual invocations.

The power of prayer in dieting and weight loss may seem odd— or even unbelievable to some—but it is based on a principle that has long been central to programs such as Alcoholics Anonymous and other 12-step programs that work on seemingly uncontrollable urges. They have this unifying concept: if you have a higher power, give yourself over to it.

Research confirms the power of prayer. In a study published in the *Journal of the American Medical Association*, researchers asked an interesting question. Who would lose more weight: women in a traditional weight-loss group or women in a faith-based weight-loss group? The experimental period was 12 weeks long.

Fifty-nine overweight and obese women were assigned to one of two groups. One was a weight-loss group that involved getting together to discuss diet tools to help them lose weight. The other was a faith-based weight-loss group that incorporated prayer and a scripture each week into the group discussion. For example, in week 6, 1 Corinthians 6:12 was chosen to underscore the fact that individuals may choose a variety of foods but that some foods are less healthful:

"'I have the right to do anything,' you say—but not everything is beneficial" (New International Version Bible).

The results of this study were interesting. Basically the women in the faith-based program lost more weight, and much of the weight was fat, as opposed to muscle. The researchers called their results "promising." I do think the addition of prayer certainly optimized these women's weight-loss experience.

While beginning my daily practice each morning, I say my morning prayer. It goes something like this:

> To the Spirit of Life, I'm yours. To build, direct, and do with me
>   as is good.
> I let go of pride and ego—I hope to do what I am meant to do.
>   I let go.
> Help me deflect roadblocks of fear and be honest, always.
> My word is good and compassionate.
> I let love and peace guide me.

Or you might try a prayer that goes something like this:

> Dear God, I desire with all my heart to stop eating so much.
> I no longer want to be under bondage to my weight problem.
> I want to live as you want me to live, free of self-destructive
>   habits and behaviors.
> I put my life into your hands, knowing that through your power
>   all things are possible.
> Strengthen me in all the weak moments. Direct my steps.
>   Change me into the kind of person who can experience
>   health, energy, and joy.
> Help me release old thoughts or old patterns of ill health and lay
>   hold of new patterns of health.
> Thank you God for renewing my mind and healing my
>   emotional needs and desires so that I run to you and not to
>   food or anything to else to satisfy me. Amen.

There are many ways to pray. You can pray for thanksgiving for the body God gave you, for self-control, or for health. Regularly practicing prayer can help calm your critical mind and can give you a more reverent and powerful experience of your body and your whole being.

Affirmations

Sometimes the easiest way to do your daily practice is to just sit in your sacred space and read passages or affirmations that are meaningful to you. Affirmations are short statements that gently reprogram your subconscious mind for success, and I offer many examples throughout this book.

We have about 25,000 to 50,000 thoughts per day, and most of those thoughts run on auto-pilot. The problem for a great many people is that so many of their thoughts are set on worry—even if this worry is not warranted. So affirmations, used correctly, can help restore you to the opposite of worry—calm.

It's helpful when you are getting started to use prewritten affirmations. Once you understand how to write them, your own affirmations will be much more powerful. When they are self-written, affirmations become much more personal and, therefore, much more effective.

Here's a lesson in how to write your own affirmations.

1. Affirmations should evoke strong emotions within you, such as excitement, happiness, or joy. If they do not bring out any positive feelings, then they are not powerful enough and you should look at changing one or two words to see if that change evokes any good feelings. If your affirmation brings out negative emotions, then you need to start over.

2. Be specific in your wording, and try to get to the heart of your challenge. For instance, if you were to say, "I am thin and light," this may immediately bring up negative mind chatter and you may hear that little voice inside of your head saying, "That's not true . . . you are not thin or light!"

    Instead, make the affirmation more true to your life. For example, "I am on my way to thin and light."

3. Be clear about the purpose of the affirmation. There's no sense in using an affirmation to boost your morale when really you are struggling with your weight. So identify what area in your life you want to work on. This will help you to write more specific, focused, and powerful affirmations. Example: "I am beautiful today, even as I claim my thinner and healthier future."

4. Affirmations are, by definition, positive. Phrase your affirmations in the positive, focusing on what you want to happen, instead of what you don't want to happen. If you write, "I don't want to be fat," you will focus on being fat—that is just how the mind works. Instead say, "I am healthy and have a *beautiful* body," "I happily choose healthy foods," "I feel great when I exercise," or, "I am becoming slimmer and healthier every day, and I feel great!" Again, phrase everything positively.

After you have identified some areas for improvement and written out your affirmations, use them in your daily practice. Speak them aloud as a chant, if you want. This works well because your body has the sensation of speaking, feeling, and hearing the words as you say them, and your feelings are engaged by those sensations.

Listen to how the statements make you feel. Do they make you feel excited, happy, uplifted, or some other positive emotion? Powerful, effective affirmations will evoke all these positive emotions, and more.

In my 30-Day Action Plan, I provide you with 30 daily affirmations to be used as you wish.

Nightly Gratitude

What you think about before you go to bed can determine your course of action the next day. As you lie down to sleep each night, think about three to five things in your life for which you have gratitude or thankfulness. They can be very simple. In my own nightly gratitude, I might say, "I am grateful my dog loves me. I am grateful I have taken good care of myself today. I am grateful my parents are in my life today. I am grateful that I have some hair on my head. I am grateful I have food in the cupboard."

Try this each night for at least three weeks. By the end of that time, you may notice that you are approaching life differently, looking for the things that fill you with that positive sense of gratitude.

There is always gratitude to be found, I promise you. Even on my darkest days, I found gratitude, and it helped me enormously. A friend calls it "the attitude of gratitude," while my great-grandma Coleman called it finding "good in the bad." Today these nightly gratitudes are part of my everyday life.

Give Step 3 a Chance to Work in Your Life!

"I don't believe this will work for me," my childhood friend Vickie told me in a huff. I'd challenged her to adopt a daily practice, but she found it confusing and scary. Vickie spent very little quality time with herself, so I just knew it could help her.

Vickie's life was so frenetic, mostly preoccupied with dieting. You name the diet craze, she was on it: the Cookie Diet, the Master Cleanse, the Bacon Diet. A perky blonde from Southern California, Vickie had once been prescribed Fen-phen; and then, after that medication was yanked off the market because it could kill you, she switched back to the latest food craze. Vickie also got liposuction on several self-described "problem areas."

Nothing worked. No solution lasted. Gradually, Vickie added weight to her 135-pound frame, but she didn't notice it right away. "My clothes were getting tighter, but I thought they were shrinking in the wash," she told me. Over the next three years, Vickie gained 55 pounds, and her weight rose to 190 pounds. She chain-smoked, too, and wheezed and coughed. Vickie was just miserable. Her face thickened and her spirit fogged over. Still, Vickie packed on more weight to her once-thin frame.

One night, Vickie decided to sleep in her boyfriend's extra-large T-shirt and found that it fit snugly in spots. "It shocked me that his 6-foot-1 clothes were tight on me," she said. "I knew I had to get my eating under control."

SLEEP AND RENEWAL

Is your bed making you fat?

Medical studies performed in the past few years are revealing that sleep loss can contribute to weight gain. It interferes with our circadian rhythms and with the regulation of hormones.

There are two hormones that affect the appetite: leptin and ghrelin. Leptin communicates that full feeling and, when everything is working correctly, suppresses appetite. Ghrelin communicates the need for more food to keep energy levels up.

When you don't get enough sleep, both hormones are thrown out of whack. Leptin goes down, making you feel less satisfied even when you've had enough food, and ghrelin goes up, stimulating your appetite.

So, what can you do to avoid sleep-related weight gain? Here are some suggestions for achieving a better night's sleep as well as a healthier lifestyle.

- Wind down before bedtime doing something relaxing, such as taking a bath.

I again pleaded with Vickie to develop a daily practice and commit to a food plan. I knew it would help her consciously surrender some of the control of her eating and dieting behavior with quietness, intention, and focus.

At the end of her physical and emotional rope, she agreed (finally) to try it. I helped her see that she could embrace a daily practice that reflected her Christian faith. She eventually added meditation and yoga. All of it helped her focus on each day with a positive attitude.

Vickie admitted to me that adopting a daily practice had been transformative. "I guess I had been searching for something more spiritual in my life, something that made me feel more at peace

- Go to bed and get up at the same time every day. Keeping consistent bedtimes and wake-up times all week is important.

- For better sleep, avoid caffeine after 5 P.M., alcohol in general, and exercise right before going to bed.

- Enjoy fish in your diet at least three times weekly. The healthy fats in fish help normalize leptin levels.

- Try relaxation techniques while in bed, such as tensing and releasing your toes, then toes and calves, and so on all the way up your body until you feel completely stress-free.

- Make sure your room is dark, cool, clean, and quiet to induce sleep. Close your curtains completely and shut the doors to the TV armoire at night or cover the TV with a scarf or towel.

- Choose a color for your bedroom that is soothing rather than stimulating; this helps the energy in your bedroom support relaxation and sleep.

- If you are still lying in bed and finding it difficult to get to sleep, try breathing slowly and deeply for 20 breaths or so.

within myself, something that let me tune in and love myself more. This new habit has a very positive effect on my physical, mental, and emotional well-being."

Vickie's food habits were tied in to her nicotine habit and both were so wrapped up in her routines that she feared if she were to stop smoking, she'd gain even more weight. I encouraged her to tackle it as I had, and as so many others I've worked with have. Don't dance with it—tackle it. Quit smoking now. You can do it, and it will increase the effectiveness of your *Just 10* plan.

Outcome studies show that those who start a change plan with food or alcohol or drugs and also quit smoking at the same time have a higher rate of success over time. Why? Tobacco strengthens the effects of the release of chemicals in the brain caused by food, which intensifies food cravings for the smoker. Here are some proven strategies to quit smoking:

1. Set a stop date, and tell those around you that you've made the decision to quit.

2. Use a nicotine replacement therapy like Nicoderm or Commit lozenges for a step-down process over several weeks.

3. Accept support from family and friends as you honor your lungs, heart, and whole body through quitting,

Vickie quit smoking, just like I did, and used the time she would have spent smoking in her daily practice. Soon enough, her daily practice and food plan sent her down a new, committed path. Vickie became naturally health conscious and lost the weight, and today she is living a much more serene life.

Up until now, you probably spent a lot of time thinking about not eating, which makes you obsess about food and about wishing you were thinner. You probably spent a lot of time looking at yourself and feeling bad about your appearance, which likely makes you sad and uptight. You ended up hiding out and avoiding certain activities that might actually make you feel better. In turn, you probably used food to comfort yourself.

With a positive daily practice, this negativity will lift. You'll be less obsessed with food. You'll start naturally forming better health habits. You'll free yourself from self-destructive patterns of the past. You'll start to love yourself more. All of this will produce weight loss.

Let each morning introduce you to new visions, new surprises, and new blessings on your way to becoming a much more vital and content person.

It's time to hurry up and be still.

Take 10

1. The more overstimulating your environment, the more solitude you probably need. For example, people with high-pressure jobs or who care for small children tend to require extra time alone.

2. Set aside time for you—and only you—at least once a day. If you have children or multiple jobs, this may be difficult to pull off. But when you do, you reap immeasurable rewards.

3. Make a commitment to use this daily practice as your own stepping-stone to a healthier, happier, and thinner life.

4. Begin with 5 to 10 minutes a day.

5. Once you're comfortable with that, increase your time to 20 minutes. After a few weeks to a few months, you should notice that you're calmer and less reactive.

6. Do your daily practice at the same time every day. Establishing a routine trains the mind to anticipate relaxation at a certain time.

7. Listen to soothing sounds that don't have a melody, lyrics, or beat.

8. Consider aromatherapy to add to the mood. It can aid in relaxation and focus. Lavender, rosemary, sandalwood, clary sage, rose, frankincense, and pine are good choices.

9. Use breathing to calm you down. Close your eyes. Focus on your heart and lungs. Slow your breath. Breathe in for a count of three, lightly hold for a count of three, and exhale slowly all the way out for a count of three. Breathe in deeply, using your diaphragm. Do this five or six times. Now allow your breath to go back to its natural rhythm.

10. Place personal troubles and the pressures of life as far away as possible, and think about having a perfectly healthy day. It will help if you turn off your iPhone or BlackBerry during this time of reflection.

JUST 10 **MYTH BUSTER**
ALL STRESS IS BAD

Stress is understandably blamed for a lot of things: fatigue, heart disease, high blood pressure. Too much stress should be avoided at all costs. But a growing number of health professionals are claiming that some stress isn't a one-way ticket to illness and an early grave. In fact, a little bit of short-term stress can actually benefit the immune system and the aging process. I know—it's hard to believe.

A Bristol University study of 5,600 men in 27 workplaces in Scotland found a lower incidence of heart disease and death overall in those most likely to say their lives were stressful. Scientists believe that if your body is stressed, it is stimulated; and therefore it continually has its immunological defenses tested and provoked, which strengthens it.

But it's the degree and duration of stress that are crucial. Short-term stress is what helps you write your best report, ace your tennis game, and meet deadlines. Long-term stress—severe and enduring stress brought on by things such as caring for someone with a long illness or living in a bad marriage or primary relationship—is harmful for most of the body's systems and can lead to physical and emotional health problems, including weight gain.

Chronic stress tells your body to keep churning out the hormone cortisol, causing you to continually reach for sugary and fat-laden foods. And cortisol signals your body to store fat, particularly at your middle.

You can use several of the steps in this program to create a stress-control prescription that's just right for your mind, body, and spirit.

CHAPTER FOUR

| STEP 4 | Appreciate Your Body |

've never been to a nudist resort—and, frankly the notion scares me a little bit—but my friends Jerry and Kura have. I quizzed them about it. I wanted to discover what lessons they gained by taking it all off. They told me the experience is not about walking around naked and looking at other naked bodies. It's about feeling contented in your own skin, literally.

The resort, said my friends, was a sea of real bodies, saggy boobs and bellies, people of all ages and in all different shapes and sizes. As their trip progressed, they became more and more comfortable with being naked, and they sure didn't miss the pressure of picking out something to wear every morning. But most of all, they found themselves feeling less critical about their own bodies—and increasingly health-conscious in a peaceful, sensible way.

I know what you're probably thinking. If you're like me, the thought of walking around naked even at a health club isn't easy. And at a nude beach? Forget about it!

I'm not recommending a weekend of nudity to make you like your body more, but I am suggesting that if you can get to a similar psychological place—feeling comfortable in your body—you will have taken a huge leap toward losing the next pound, reaching your ideal weight, and restoring a positive relationship with your body.

When you like your body and consistently treat it with respect, you will lose weight—and never gain it back. This is what Step 4 is all about.

How Much Do You Like Your Body?

Please answer these 10 questions with a "yes" or "no" response. Be honest. No one is looking.

1. Do you hate to look at yourself in mirrors when you pass by them?
Yes ☐ No ☐

2. Are you uncomfortable lying naked in front of someone with whom you're intimate?
Yes ☐ No ☐

3. Do you feel conspicuous wearing a bathing suit in public?
Yes ☐ No ☐

4. Do you often wear baggy clothes that hide your size?
Yes ☐ No ☐

5. Do you look in the mirror and focus only on the neck up?
Yes ☐ No ☐

6. Do you often avoid buying clothes because of how they look?
Yes ☐ No ☐

7. If someone stares at you when you walk by, do you feel conscious of your appearance?
Yes ☐ No ☐

8. Do you often discount compliments on your appearance, brushing them off and saying, "Oh, I look horrible"?
Yes ☐ No ☐

9. Do you dislike parts of your body, such as your thighs or belly?

Yes ☐ No ☐

10. Do you tend to negatively compare yourself to other people who you think are thinner or better-looking than you?

Yes ☐ No ☐

Scoring: Score a point for each "yes" answer.

8 or more: You don't like your body or appearance very much. You've got work to do, and this step will help you.

4 to 7: You're borderline. It's time to call a truce. Enlist the easy body-loving strategies in this step.

2 to 3: You have a healthy respect for your body. Look at the questions for which you answered "yes." These are areas for improvement.

0 or 1: Congratulations! You seem at peace with your body. But don't stop nurturing it now. Continue to treat your body well and use kind words when you're talking about it. It'll repay you by looking and feeling good.

The Five Body Hang-ups and How to Overcome Them

Many of us are living with body hatred. We detest the way we look. But why? How did it get to be this way? Why do we moan about our bodies each time we look in the mirror? Why do we say, "Oh my God, I want to look like that" when we leaf through a magazine? Why in our private conversations with ourselves are we so brutal, not telling ourselves how wonderful and beautiful we are, but rather how bad, ugly, and helpless we are? And why have we come to accept this body hatred as unavoidably the way things are and will remain?

One way of answering these questions is to take a look at the origins of body hatred. In this step, I'll drag some monsters out into the light—what I call the five body hang-ups—so we can stare them down before overcoming them. Take a close look at each point in this step, without self-judgment. Just read with compassion and honesty, and note how many of these things you have experienced or you have done to yourself. Awareness is the beginning of renewing a positive relationship with your body.

Overcoming Body Hang-up #1:
Outgrow Family Pressure

When we're kids—when our faces haven't grown into our noses, when we haven't shed our baby fat, when we get zits, when our breasts develop (or don't develop as the case may be), when we're too short or too gangly—is when our body image takes form and stays with us into adulthood.

Body image is not just that visual image we hold in our mind's eye, but also the feelings and thoughts we have in response to that image. I know it sounds simple, but if you don't like your body, you are apt not to like yourself much. By contrast, if you like and accept your looks, it is much easier to like and accept yourself. And when you appreciate "you," the by-product is a beautiful, healthy body.

Yet as grown-ups, many of us still perceive ourselves as overweight, lumbering, or otherwise unattractive, the same way we felt during our childhood or teen years. You may have been brought up in a family in which there was a particular emphasis on appearance, or you may have family members who were slim and with whom you were unfavorably compared. Some of the harshest and most frequent ribbing over appearance occurs at home and comes from siblings and parents. Many women with body hatred had mothers who badgered them about their bodies when they were younger, and they do it to themselves as adults. I hear stories of girls who sat on Daddy's lap and heard, "God, you sure got fat! You're not my little girl anymore." In a study conducted in part by Harvard Medical School, teenage girls who said their parents made comments about their weight were more than twice as likely as their peers to be highly concerned about their body image one year later.

Anecdotally, I can tell you that the sting of body-related criticism tends to linger for longer than a year. If a family member has ever told you you're fat, chances are you've never forgotten it. Joanie, a client of mine, sure didn't. Twenty years ago a "lighthearted" observation by her father triggered a dieting lifestyle that lasted a decade.

Joanie elaborated: "I wasn't really fat, maybe eight or nine pounds overweight. He said, 'You're as big as Aunt Lilly's house,' when I returned home from college. I was crushed. I immediately vowed to stop eating until I lost weight." Those words set off an extreme reaction in Joanie that triggered years of yo-yo dieting and self-loathing.

Another client remembers sitting on her grandmother's lap in grade school, just after she'd experienced a growth spurt and began developing breasts. Her grandmother exclaimed she'd gotten "too fat to sit on my lap!" She recalled an odd tension, feeling wrong and ashamed by it. She felt her body had turned against her, resulting in the loss of something she loved—being physically close, in a lovely way, with her grandmother.

If relatives' negative comments about your body are still with you today, understand that, while their messages may have been poorly expressed, their true intention was for you to grow up to be healthy and happy. Forgive your relatives—we're all imperfect beings—and take a realistic look at the part of your body that you felt they improperly criticized.

Let go of the past, forgive, and take time out of your everyday life to invest in yourself and your health. You cannot explore new frontiers if you are holding on to the old ones. Do what it takes to release the shackles of your past and move on.

Keep in mind, too, that what others think of you is none of your business. It's not your issue. (More on this in Chapter 5.) You are responsible only for what you think of yourself, so make it positive.

Overcoming Body Hang-up #2:
Remember Beauty is in the Eye of the Beholder

Some of you may work in environments in which there are intense pressures to be slim, such as in dance, modeling, or entertainment. I understand. I was a weather anchor on the TV news; and trust me, there was tremendous pressure to stay in shape and have perfect hair, skin, and teeth. If someone told me I was getting pudgy or I needed a better haircut, it was tough to take. I didn't feel good about myself. It was so personal and incredibly rude, even if it was the nature of the business.

We live in an appearance-conscious culture. Women are reminded to be sleek, sexy, and slim; men must be muscular, sexy, and trim. Yet few of us naturally possess such physiques. We're ordinary mortals; and we've got bulges, folds, fat, and fleshiness. That's just life, and it isn't going to change anytime soon. The sooner we realize that the world doesn't revolve around the appearance of our asses, tummies, boobs, and thighs, the better!

There's no empirical standard of beauty, anyway. It's in the eye of the beholder, remember? Besides, in some eras, a Rubinesque woman was greatly appreciated, and in some cultures, a larger body size is a sign of status. So to get over this hang-up, realize that opinions on beauty change greatly, believe you're beautiful, and take care of yourself accordingly. True beauty comes from many places: It radiates from confidence, quiet seriousness, and feelings of happiness and passion. It comes from staying true to yourself, keeping your head high, not caring what others think, smiling, and showing bravery and hopefulness. To be truly beautiful, *you have to believe* that you are beautiful. Nothing can change that, and nothing ever will. And if you believe you're beautiful, other people will believe it, too.

There's something so appealing about people who move through space feeling good about themselves. None of us has the "perfect body" (there is no such thing, anyway) but people are attracted to confidence in others. I'm not referring to arrogance, but rather self-contentment.

Another powerful tool for overcoming body hatred is to wear clothes that make you feel beautiful. I'm not talking about baggy stuff that just happens to feel comfortable. No, I'm talking about clothes that show off your best parts: a great bustline, shapely calves, a small waist—whatever you like best. These are clothes that you feel good in. And as your budget allows, invest in more outfits that make you feel wonderful.

And while I'm on the subject, throw out your fat clothes! As soon as you drop a dress or pants size, don't be tempted to keep the clothes that no longer fit. You can rationalize this as hanging on to clothes in case you ever need them again, but really, it's just setting yourself up for failure. Get rid of that Emergency Clothes Reserve Unit! Get rid of it. And don't you dare buy clothes that are bigger than you need because you don't believe you will keep the weight off. Have faith, conviction, and certainty that you will be slim and fit forever.

My closet used to be divided in two. There were fat clothes and thin clothes. Once I met my weight goal, I went through my closet, weeded out all of the clothes that were too big, and gave them to charity. This was such a huge step for me—an incredible act of self-love.

Be positive that you won't regain the weight and don't look back.

Overcoming Body Hang-up #3: Learn the New Math on Beauty Ideals

We buy into society's messages that say there should be less of us. Messages about the "perfect" body type—unattainable for the vast majority of us—are so pervasive that even younger kids can't escape them, and this is why plastic surgery among kids and teens is on the upswing. We wildly underestimate the extent to which we succumb to media influences—billboards, fashion ads, movie images, and cell phone promotions—and start to assume and incorporate these notions of truth and beauty into our own opinions of ourselves.

If you're vulnerable to this hang-up, I suggest a reality check. The average American woman is 5 feet 4 inches tall and weighs 140 pounds, while the average American model is 5 feet 11 inches tall and weighs 117 pounds, making her thinner than 98 percent of American women. So mathematically, it would be pointless to judge your body in terms of someone you have only a 2 percent genetic possibility of looking like. Math doesn't lie.

We also compare ourselves to our own relatives and our best friends. If you compare yourself to anyone you think has a better body than yours, this can become a dangerous mind trip.

Instead, work on comparing yourself to you. Focus on your life-affirming and totally doable *Just 10* weight-loss goal. I'm with you on it and know you can make it! Commit to taking care of your body in ways that make you feel sexier and stronger. Try yoga, do your moving meditation, or go to the gym. Work on improving yourself to create a better, healthier version of yourself, a picture of yourself at a healthy weight that you can achieve—not an impossible one guaranteed to bring on disappointment. Conjure a self-image goal. It could be a mental snapshot from the past—such as when you were a size 6 before having kids—or one that reveals a realistic future. Remember, too, it's best if the image is in motion and illustrates how your body's abilities are improving. For example, try visualizing yourself in a yoga pose that you're able to do because of your newfound flexibility.

Overcoming Body Hang-up #4: Revel in Physical Distinctiveness

Some of us attract more negative attention than others because our appearance is distinctive in some way. For example, I didn't like who I saw in the mirror because I had developed abnormal breasts in grade school. That's right—breasts. I was born with a birth defect: developing breast tissue. As a boy, I looked like I needed a bra, even though, at that point, I wasn't a fat kid.

In fifth grade, I was exposed to a coach who took delight in making sure I was always a "skin"; that is, assigned to the team that had to take their shirts off to play ball. "Look at Lamm's tits!" the coach would yell. It was cruel. The other kids teased me. I refused to take a shower at school after gym class and did all I could to keep my secret. I wrapped tape around my chest and then bundled up with a tight T-shirt under a loose sweater. I felt ashamed of my body. I told my parents I wanted to kill myself.

My crisis forced a decision on their part—to correct my deformity as soon as possible. At age 15, I had surgery, courtesy of a physician aptly named Dr. Cutler; and voilà, the outside had changed. Yes, the physical problem was improved, fixed. But the psychological scars of being laughed at and mocked as a kid still remained. I tried to remove the scars with food, alcohol, and drugs, but I still hated living in my own body.

Being too short or too tall, or having acne or any distinctive feature, may result in unwanted attention or teasing from others. We tend to internalize the taunts and make them another reason to dislike ourselves.

Instead, why not make your unusual features your calling card, your personal insignia? It's never been easier to do this, because our current culture is much more accepting of different kinds of beauty than it was a generation ago. Individuality and character are prized, too, not just conventional good looks. Pick out your most unique feature, and then turn the spotlight on it. Do you have a mole on your face like Cindy Crawford? Show it off! A space between your two front teeth like Madonna? Play it up with some bright red lipstick. Whatever your most distinctive attribute—bristly black eyelashes or untamable hair—turn it into an intoxicating trademark. Think of Phyllis Diller, or even Troy Polamalu, the NFL player who hasn't cut his hair in 10 years and is proud of his mane. His hair was even insured for a cool $1 million because it's the hallmark of shampoo advertisements. Flaunt what you've got and never apologize for not looking like whoever the hot model of the moment is.

Overcoming Body Hang-up #5: Can the Body Spam

I refer to the negative dialogue we have with ourselves (for example, "My butt is too big" or "I hate the beauty mark on my cheek") as body spam, or unsolicited junk. These racing thoughts build on one another and can erode the foundation of how we view ourselves. And the way we talk to ourselves becomes the way we view ourselves. It's difficult to love your body when you're motivated by this sort of negativity.

BODY APPRECIATION EXERCISE
CREATE A BODY MAP

If you were asked to draw a picture of yourself, there's every chance the result would look more like Shrek than a Barbie doll. It doesn't necessarily matter if you're as skinny as a bean pole—our own sense of body image is so powerful that what you think you look like often bears little resemblance to the reality.

Early in my career of working with people with food problems, I couldn't get my head around the idea that thin people thought they were fat, and people who were quite large imagined themselves as much larger. So I employ an exercise called "Body Map."

Creating your very own Body Map is a critical exercise in helping you feel comfortable in your own skin, improve your body image, and connect your sense of self to reality. Here's how it works:

- Take a giant piece of paper (use several taped together if necessary) and draw an outline of what you believe your shape is: head, arms, breasts, hips, legs, the whole thing.

Imagine if you went around and talked to everybody that you met in terms of his or her physical faults: "Hi, Big Butt! Hello, Mr. Baldy! Good day, Love Handles!" You'd be the loneliest person in the world, assuming you survived even the first day. You wouldn't take it if someone else did that to you, right? Yet this is exactly the way we address ourselves all the time.

Think about it! When you constantly put down your body with a certain phrase (for example, "I'm a blob"), that belief becomes imprinted in your brain, so you actually begin to move like you *are* a blob. The information sinks in and becomes hard to shake.

You've got to learn to be more accepting and talk to yourself in an affectionate, loving way—and bring loving beliefs to the

- Lie over the image, or stand up against it if you can tape it to the wall, and have someone trace the real outline around you.

- Look at the two outlines. What you'll discover is that your imagined body is much different than your actual one. Write down words and feelings around different body parts. Write down years and instances, denote memories and hurts—triumphs and body tragedies. Make your map! This will help you realize what you've been feeling about your body and help you discover what's real and what's imagined. Or while you may believe that your proportions are all wrong, in fact, you may see that there's balance to your shape and beauty to your bends.

Most people are amazed by this exercise, because they don't look anything like they think they do. Find more info on Body Mapping in your *Just 10 Workbook*, including seeing some Body Map samples that will be helpful to your work. This exercise helps you put aside your hang-ups and appreciate what's real.

forefront of your thinking. When you do that, your brain perceives and acts on these new positive beliefs as if they are already in place.

For starters, spend time thinking about how much you *like* certain aspects of your body and why you appreciate them. To be at peace with my own body, I went through practically every body part and appreciated it for what it did for me. For example:

- **My ears.** I take pleasure in listening to people talk, being a good listener, and focusing on the sounds of nature.

- **My hands.** I have long fingers that I use to make beautiful music while I'm playing the piano.

- **My legs.** I appreciate my legs. I use them for bicycling, playing soccer, and dancing. They are strong and good and get me to where I am going.

- **My voice.** I use it to communicate and to teach and inspire people who are hurting.

- **My eyes.** I love reading. I enjoy watching performances. I love to study art. Seeing my friends, my family, and my pets is the best part of my day. I love staring up at big buildings or glancing down at pretty flowers. My camera goes everywhere so I can take lots of pictures of things that fascinate me. With my eyes, I get to see all things beautiful in life.

- **My nose.** It's got a bump that sets me apart from others. It lets me enjoy and remember pleasant aromas. The list of my favorite smells could go on and on: recently mown grass in the spring, pine-scented candles at the holidays, and the smells of barbecuing nearby.

- **My skin.** I love my skin. It's pale and healthy, especially on my arms where I look at it all the time. I protect it from extremes of temperature and drink plenty of water to keep it supple and elastic.

I can sum up Step 4 in two words: Golden Rule. You know the one: treat other folks the way you'd like to be treated. Now reframe the Golden Rule like this: I will treat my body as I like to be treated: luxuriously, with love and compassion, and with the same or better kindness I show to everyone else.

Take 10

1. Boost your body image by appreciating your body for what it can do no matter what your size or shape. Try to notice how you use your body to do helpful things— for example, score a goal or carry an elderly neighbor's

groceries—instead of treating it as an object to be looked at judgmentally. Love all the good things your body does for you.

2. If body spam creeps into your thinking, immediately replace hurtful insults with a phrase that captures a nonbody-related trait you love about yourself; for example, "I am confident" or "I am a loving friend." You may not believe your new phrase immediately, but over time you can convince yourself to be more positive.

3. Make a deal with yourself that every time you say something bad about your body ("My thighs are so huge"), you have to wipe it out with a strong positive statement ("My thighs feel so good when I'm biking").

4. If you've lost weight, people will comment that you look good. Take these compliments to heart. Don't push them away with something like, "You need to have your eyes checked."

5. Think about things you excel in, such as hobbies or work projects.

6. Write down the daily commitments you make toward losing weight in your journal or *Just 10 Workbook*. This exercise will help you feel more positive about your body because you have a sense of accomplishment. Your list might include such things as taking long walks, eating extra veggies, and drinking eight glasses of water each day.

7. Make friends with your full-length mirror. This isn't easy, but the more you look, the less you'll stress.

8. Sleep naked. Going to bed with absolutely nothing between you and the sheets is one way to reconnect you with, and to love, your body. In fact, getting accustomed to being in the buff is a significant step toward feeling really good in your own skin. So toss

out the old sweatpants and oversized T-shirts for good. It's a sexy or slightly naughty secret, and a great boost to your confidence.

9. Your moving meditation is key to loving your body; do it because it feels good, not as a dieting strategy.

10. Be patient with yourself. You didn't develop your negative body image overnight, so don't expect an instant turnaround.

JUST 10 MYTH BUSTER
BODY-IMAGE DISTORTION IS ONLY A PROBLEM FOR WOMEN

Body-image problems are typically seen in women, but many men have problems, too, particularly some athletes. Case in point: for bodybuilders, getting big and muscular consumes their lives—a preoccupation with muscular appearance known as "body dysmorphia." Those with the disorder feel they're not big enough, despite the fact that they're quite large and fit. Classic symptoms of body dysmorphia include deliberate overtraining, overdieting, using steroids to build muscle despite known adverse consequences, and giving up social activities and occupations that you'd normally enjoy because you don't like your physical condition or because you're afraid the activity will disrupt your fitness schedule.

CHAPTER FIVE

STEP 5 Love Yourself Thin

M any of my clients eat the way I used to eat. They're compulsive bingers, not because they're legitimately hungry, but because they're emotionally hungry. Some have suffered overweight-related diseases and spent years trying to reboot their eating routines. Their lives are chaos central, due to food.

What's the answer? We all must learn to love ourselves enough to make better choices. This is what Step 5 is all about: learning to love yourself.

What does it mean to love yourself? I've asked this question to groups, and everyone offers a different opinion. Among the top definitions: self-respect, confidence, keeping your body healthy, and believing in your own possibilities.

I know what self-love is not: feeling that you never want to be who you are. You never look at yourself and say, "I'm the best I can be." Instead, you look and say, "I don't like me."

If you don't love yourself, life will always be hard to live.

I call self-love "Dramamine for the soul." When the waves of life rock our world, self-love keeps us from getting sick.

Let me get more specific. As a working definition, *self-love* is any action we take for our physical, mental, and spiritual enhancement. The following are some examples of self-love.

- I eat body-honoring foods.

- I take care of my body and my health.

- I do my moving meditation.

- I don't ignore my needs at the expense of others.

- I've shed the need for approval or recognition. I am not who others think I should be.

- I focus on my body's assets, rather than its liabilities.

- I avoid self-criticism.

- I concentrate on where I am now and where I want to go.

- I reward and praise myself after any and all achievements.

- I focus on my strengths, not on my weaknesses.

- I love my body and everything it does for me.

- I'm assertive when necessary.

- I express my feelings, opinions, beliefs, and needs directly, openly, and honestly, but without violating the rights of others.

- I do not judge others.

- I view myself as a winner who sees every circumstance, good or bad, as an opportunity.

- I believe I deserve to have what I want.

- I don't procrastinate; I know that accomplishment is the result of activity.

- I accept winning as a natural and inevitable state of events.

- I value the spiritual side of life.

- I experience joyful days.

Yes, this is a long list of self-loving actions. But if you're enacting even a couple of points on this list, you're doing great! The more you can add over time, the better.

So let's talk about how to do that.

Start Loving Yourself Today

The journey of self-love follows a crazed, twisted, bumpy road. If you're now thinking, *I don't have time to go down that road,* don't worry, it won't take long. That's one of the beautiful things about this step. It's so simple. Once you apply it, you'll gain great insight into yourself, and you'll suddenly understand why you've been acting and reacting the way you have. You'll now be able to work with your own thoughts and feelings to move yourself forward.

No matter how bad, down, or crappy you feel right now, start acting as if you love yourself. Sometimes you have to fake it before it becomes the real deal. Acting means you take on the mind-set of what you wish to become and allow (or encourage) your behaviors to follow. If you practice long enough, your acting is no longer acting. It's real.

In your daily practice, the first priority of your day is loving yourself. Self-love is most effective if you practice it every day rather than waiting for the right time. Affirm throughout the day that you love yourself. Notice the huge difference it makes as you go about your day.

From there, practice loving yourself with simple actions. Pamper yourself with little things every day. Snuggle up with a cup of tea or curl up with a favorite book or magazine. Settle into a tub of bubbles or put on your favorite music. Pick up a flower at the grocery store so that every time you look at it you will smile. Light candles in your home or put crystals in the window so that rainbows dance across your room. These always make me smile.

Decide for yourself that you are indeed worth loving. This is a "just do it" kind of thing, not something you can do merely to please your mom, your spouse, your boyfriend, your best friend, or anyone other than yourself. If it's not really for you, it just won't happen.

Declare today, "From now on, no matter how tough life may be or how imperfect I may feel, I am going to honestly love myself."

Loving Yourself Is An Inside Job

You've got to practice listening to your inner voice to discover the ways and means of achieving self-love. All too often we are our harshest critics, and we are more judgmental toward ourselves than anyone in our lives. And those thoughts are precisely what often stand in the way of achieving the things we most want in life, including a thin, healthy body. Negative dialogue is unproductive, hinders success (at anything), and is the prime means of harboring hopelessness. Positive dialogue, on the other hand, produces the exact opposite: hopefulness. Change starts within, and what better place to address negativity than in our head and heart?

Unlocking the Secret to Self-Love

In my workshops and sessions with clients, I ask people where their lack of self-love comes from. Most everyone says it originally developed from their parents; the way they were raised; and influences, good and bad, from their varied life experiences. The doubt and self-loathing also come from inflated feelings, skewed perceptions, and incorrect self-reporting.

Certainly all of these things and many more are part of the answer. We're a product of vivid hurt-generating events from the past, especially from childhood, perhaps including emotional, physical, and/or sexual abuse; domineering coaches; negativity-spouting relatives; and controlling significant others (to name a few). Lack of self-love comes from many corners, and it almost always resonates as hurtful feelings that we carry around with us.

But there is also something much more significant that is often completely missed: *the questions we ask ourselves.*

We're constantly asking ourselves questions such as, *What is he thinking of me? How do I look in this dress? How do I fit in here? What should I do in this situation? How will this affect the outcome?* The questions we ask ourselves generate all kinds of thoughts, some positive, some negative. It's the negative thoughts that don't serve us well. They slowly chip away at our self-love.

Let me give you an example of how one question could be in conflict with the relationship you have with yourself, and how it could derail you on your quest for greater self-love.

One of the dominant questions people allow to knock around in their heads is "What are they thinking of me?" The primary problem with this question is that it puts other people in the driver's seat of your life. While a question like this might motivate you to get other people to think good things about you, you can never know for sure what other people are thinking. And, most important, do you really want to base your life on what other people think of you?

There is a story about Buddha. One day while teaching a group of people, Buddha met a man who was angered by Buddha's teachings. The angry man kept insulting him and criticizing him at every turn.

Finally Buddha turned to the man and said, "If someone offers you a gift but you choose to decline it, tell me, who would then own the gift?"

The man said, "It belongs to the giver. Any fool can see that."

Buddha smiled. "That is correct. So if I decline to accept abuse, does it not still belong to you?"

The man was speechless and walked away.

The point is: it doesn't matter what others think about me or my actions, so I don't even ask myself that question. What others think about me is none of my business. And, it's not all about me; people are wrapped up in their own lives, and rarely are we occupying the kind of prime real estate in their brains that we imagine we are.

When you love yourself, your happiness never depends on what others think of you, on how impressive your job/house/friends are to the rest of the world, or on how many presents you get on your birthday. Self-love is an inside job.

If this sounds like a lot of New Age nonsense, it's not. When you learn to love yourself, you have the confidence to survive disapproval, should it occur. You know deep in your bones that you can't possibly please all of the people all of the time, and so you come to understand that occasionally you will disappoint and upset others. The more you trust yourself and assert your autonomy, the more your love will come from a genuine place in your heart, rather than from some compulsion to please, avoid confrontation, or keep peace.

All of this stems from the questions we ask ourselves. If you can control the questions you ask yourself, you can begin to consciously change the way you feel about yourself, love yourself more, and ultimately change your circumstances. So ask questions that lead to positive, productive, and action-oriented thinking.

The questions we ask ourselves fall into two categories: loving questions and unloving questions.

Unloving Questions

Why me? Why can't I ever lose weight? What's with this bad luck lately? Why can't I stay on a diet? Why can't I stop this terrible habit? How did I screw up so badly?

Imagine having those types of questions constantly roaming around in your mind. They make you focus on what a failure you are and how your situation seems utterly hopeless.

Continue asking unloving questions for months, years, even decades, and your whole life becomes ruled by the negative thoughts and the emotions they elicit. This can be a vicious downward spiral.

You must change your questions.

Loving Questions

Why not me? What's good about this situation that I'm probably overlooking? What actions can I take right now to improve my weight? Even though I've got some weight to lose, what am I thankful for in my life right now?

Do you see the difference between the two sets of questions? Loving questions help you find positive solutions to your situation. They give you control over a situation rather than make you a victim of it.

Questions are at the core of how we listen, behave, and relate. Virtually everything we think and do is generated by questions. Questions can push us into new territories, help us reach greater goals, and trigger positive life change. Questions are magical, but we must know how to ask the *right* questions.

Great Results Begin with Great Questions

During my first and only rehab to get off drugs and alcohol, and to get healthier with food, I thought a lot about my life, how I wanted to live, and the impact I wanted to have on the world. At first, everything I wanted seemed impossible or improbable. I didn't yet love myself enough to move forward. I had trouble even looking people in the eye, let alone asking the big question of "what's next?" I was still too ashamed of who I was.

But I learned to ask myself a lot of questions. Based on my experience as a former weather anchor and journalist, I asked myself these six questions: who, what, where, when, why, and how. I answered every question, and the answers led me to solutions. Great results begin with great questions, and the answers discovered.

Loving Questions That Will Change Your Weight and Your Life

Look over these questions; then take some time to answer them. Each question holds its answer within, so don't make it more difficult than it has to be. Let the answer develop naturally. The answers give you clarity and understanding. You'll begin to see solutions that will move you forward rather than hold you back. You'll gain flashes of insight into yourself, and you'll start to improve any "less than" thoughts you've learned and retained.

Lots of things will start to make sense: why you haven't been losing weight, why you've been procrastinating, why you feel stressed, or why you're just not accomplishing what you feel you should be by now. And, you'll not only understand yourself better, you'll also see the direction you want and need to go in.

Who

- Who can help me?
- Who can support me?
- Who can I celebrate with?

What

- What do I want?
- What are the steps to get what I want?
- What must I change?
- What do I need to do to help myself?
- What am I grateful for?
- What can I learn from this?
- What are the consequences of not changing this behavior or situation?

Where

- Where will change take me?
- Where do I find help and resources?
- Where I am now compared to where I want to be?

When

- When will I start?
- When will I get there?

Why

- Why do I want to change?
- Why is change important?

How

- How can I accomplish this?

- How have others done it?

- How do I begin to nurture myself better?

- How does continuing this behavior serve me?

Want to see how these questions work in real life? Read the following stories and discover the power of asking loving questions.

Anna's Story

Anna always considered herself a "big girl." "I weighed 9 pounds when I was born, and I was always the biggest girl in my class at school," she told me. Thanks to an unhealthy diet in high school and college, Anna stayed heavy into adulthood. By her mid-20s, Anna weighed 180 pounds at 5 feet 5 inches.

"Then I got married, and the tension of an unhappy marriage turned me into a stress eater," she admitted. Five years later, Anna's weight peaked at 275 pounds. "When I finally left my marriage, I was a mess. I was out of shape, unhealthy, and disgusted with myself."

I encouraged Anna to consider some specific questions: How does stress eating serve you? Her answer: "It calms me down temporarily, but makes me feel terrible about myself. And it's making me gain weight."

Then I asked, "What do you think will happen if you don't change this behavior?"

Anna shuddered. She didn't even want to think about it. She knew that she could be in trouble—physically, emotionally, and spiritually—if something didn't change soon.

I continued to quiz her. "What positive behaviors could calm you down—plus make you healthier?"

This line of questioning prompted Anna to develop a plan to counter her destructive stress eating. She learned to start her day with 10 minutes of peaceful reflection and self-love affirmations. She began eating according to her style. She found she enjoyed the solitude of weight training—an activity that improved her self-image, made her feel athletic, and helped her be more appreciative of her body.

Anna began to take care of herself by asking loving questions and choosing thoughts and actions that were elevating and kind. The more she believed that she is a beautiful person on the inside and worth the effort to change, the less she overate out of stress or despair.

If you don't like something you're doing—and you hate your-self for doing it anyway—ask yourself how the behavior or habit is serving you. Ask and answer that question. It will open your head and heart to healthier options that serve the same purpose. And you'll begin to engage in those behaviors. Loving questions ener-gize the process of change and self-love.

Marie's Story

If you've ever dieted unsuccessfully, you can relate to Marie. She is like a lot of people today. Marie struggles with her weight and always has—she loses 15 pounds, regains 25, loses 20, and regains 30. It's a common scenario.

"I knew it was just a matter of time before I'd lose momentum trying to lose weight," Marie told me. "I knew well the signs of self-sabotage: Too busy to get to the gym. Too bored with vegetables to keep eating them. Too exhausted from life's pressures to care."

A few months after she turned 43, 5-foot-4-inch Marie stepped on the scale and saw that she had reached an all-time high of 182 pounds. That meant that she was heavier than her 6-foot-tall, 178-pound husband.

"I was also feeling the physical effects: I couldn't cross my legs, my clothing dug into me, I felt sweaty all the time. I thought, *If I can't get my act together soon, then I never will. I can either fix myself or accept things the way they are.*"

Marie chose to fix it.

The key question Marie asked herself was, "How does a yo-yo dieter like me keep the weight off for good?"

I helped her answer this question very simply, based on her life and lifestyle. The flash-of-insight answer that emerged was: make yourself a priority!

Marie, a wife and mother of three, rarely nurtured herself. She had thoughts such as, *I don't deserve to take better care of myself.* She had fallen into the trap of thinking that taking care of her husband and kids was more important than taking care of herself. Sound familiar?

Putting herself first isn't selfish; it is a loving act. In fact, it's the best thing she could do for her family. After our work together, Marie said, "Now I have a new attitude. You know on an airplane when the flight attendant tells you to put on your own oxygen mask before you help your child or the person next to you? I feel the same way about my health. If I'm not healthy, I can't help anyone."

One question always leads to another. The other key question Marie asked was, "How do I begin to nurture myself better?"

Solutions streamed out. She committed to exercising, eating right, and taking care of her body. She began loving herself more and valuing her appearance and health.

Marie spent time every day meditating and even came up with a wonderful visualization for yo-yo dieters—a combination of chanting and visualizing.

"I said out loud, 'I'm over it, and I'm back on my plan.'" Then she'd imagine herself standing up, dusting herself off, and getting back on a horse. She'd hold that visualization for a moment and feel proud about her decision.

Marie even developed and pursued once-dormant hobbies and interests that gave her a sense of enjoyment and fulfillment. After five months, the scale hit 135 pounds and stayed there. She hadn't seen that weight since college.

And it all started with a few simple, loving questions.

My Story

There were many twists and turns in my recovery, and I'm abbreviating the story here. I knew I hadn't loved myself enough to want to get better. I had too many toxic thoughts. This all came out in further therapy when I was asked a life-changing question: "Brad, what do you think of yourself?"

My answers weren't pretty.

"I'm ugly. I'm not worth anything. I am a mess. I'm morally deficient because I'm an addict. I'm a bad person." On and on went my litany of self-disgust.

My best friend, Jerry, recalls that during this period, when I couldn't look people in the eye and was constantly in tears, he asked me what I wanted. "I want to stop crying and not die," I said. With all that lying bare, I learned to pose other questions—loving, truth-seeking questions, I call them. "Am I really worth nothing? Is it really true I'm a bad person?" I had plenty of toxic thoughts, but I had to learn how to dismiss them by asking myself these questions.

Answer: of course not! I started analyzing my own inner dialogue, dissecting it, and thinking more logically about what I was saying to myself. I was searching so hard for self-love that I never dreamed that it was hiding inside of me. The reason we have a hard time finding this love is that the clutter we have in our heads is standing in the way. When we can address this clutter, we will begin finding what we are looking for.

I carried around an incredible spiritual weight of resentment and regret—that dark resentment of self that nags and cuts and re-imagines the past in inflated and terrifying details. Along the way I learned that self-forgiveness is vital, too. It's the generous act of giving yourself a break and remembering that you're human. Self-forgiveness is a commitment to love yourself no matter what. Learning from mistakes is important, too, but mostly what we need, I believe, is less self-punishment and more self-love.

I also discovered how to use uncomfortable emotions or moods—such as stress, depression, and anxiety—as cues for listening to my self-talk. When you get in a blue mood, identify the feeling as accurately as possible. Then ask yourself, "What was I saying to myself right before I started feeling this way?" or "What have I been saying to myself since I've been feeling this way?"

Are you beginning to see the power in asking yourself the right questions? Consider what you've written down in your journal or

Just 10 Workbook around your own feelings and how you experience them. How do you feel? Are you starting to ask yourself the right questions?

With the help of therapy, I started spending more time thinking about my own strengths and talents. It can feel self-indulgent at first, but it changed my whole way of being in the world. The more I focused on my strengths, the more I started loving myself.

So I'm going to ask you to do the same. Ask yourself this loving question: "What strengths, talents, and greatness do I have?" Or put another way: "What has made me a great _____ (insert your own word: parent, husband, wife, son, daughter, employee, friend, and so forth)." Don't be shy. You have been blessed with unique talents, strengths, and abilities. Announce them to yourself!

Even if you don't immediately have all the answers, it will start you thinking about yourself in a new and positive way, instead of focusing on the gaps you believe you have to fill or the weaknesses you feel you have to overcome. This exercise—and your answers—will help you love yourself more.

If you had asked me in 2000 if this is what my life would look like now, I would have said, "No way." I've been in recovery for many years now and have the most amazing friends who love me for who I am—not for what I have or what I look like. So take it from me: by loving yourself, you get a wonderful reward—a free, happy, and healthy life. Do I love being me? You bet I do.

There are few things more important than uncovering the questions and thoughts that are controlling your life, so you can once and for all take control of your destiny.

When you start asking loving questions, you'll begin to truly love yourself. You'll come to a whole new place with food, break the cycles of crazy eating and dieting, and become ever more likely to stay at your healthy weight. Self-love was how I ultimately got control over my weight and my life, and began helping others on this same path.

So please: look within and love yourself. This is no time to throw in the towel or surrender to self-doubt. Big breakthroughs are possible. It's time to be vibrantly and vitally you.

Take 10

1. Consciously ask yourself loving questions in your daily practice. Ask yourself questions like: "What am I most happy about in my life right now?" "What am I grateful about right now?" and "What in my life is going really well for me right now?" When I ask myself these questions, here are some of the things I think about: I have a roof over my head. I'm healthy. I have people who love me. I have opportunities to help people. I live in a world where I can access information with a click of a button through the Internet. I can play the piano and write books. I have a website that reaches people all over the world.

2. Listen to your answers—big or small. The important thing is when you think about what you like about yourself and your life, be sure to really feel the associated emotions. Don't just think about them; experience them. This is powerful stuff. I get tears of joy when I do this. It can change your life as it did for me.

3. Your answers will come to you if you let them. Be clear with your intention that you are taking ownership of your present situation and crafting the solution. Remove the language of victimization from your play book. Instead of "What is life doing to me?" ask, "What is life doing for me in this moment?"

4. When you catch yourself asking unloving questions, immediately fight back. Change them into loving ones.

5. Practice asking loving questions throughout the day. If you do this over and over, it will eventually become a habit. Once that happens, you'll be able to change your focus and love yourself even more.

6. Look to and live your answers. They plot a path to powerful solutions.

7. Exercise, eat right, and take care of your body—these actions help produce self-love.

8. To love yourself, you need to learn to accept yourself the way you are: embrace yourself as a whole. Think about it: your best friend or spouse not only accepts the good and bad parts of you, but they understand why you are the way you are, and love you just the same. So be your own best friend.

9. Create self-love affirmations. Say "I love me" as often as you need to. People are more likely to stay trim if they love themselves.

10. Love yourself *no matter what.* That way, you'll take better care of your body, and the healthy changes will fall into place. Let loving behaviors toward yourself be your baseline for self-care.

JUST 10 MYTH BUSTER
SELF-LOVE IS BAD AND SELFISH

Many of us shy away from the very idea of loving ourselves. Everyone wants to be loved. But to be loved, we have to give love. And to give it, we must have it and know it for ourselves. When we overeat and treat our bodies poorly, we don't have much self-love—because we feel guilty about how much we eat and how we look. Since we don't love ourselves much, we don't act in ways that would evoke love from others, either. Moving through these steps will help you love yourself more. And when you love yourself, everything you want will fall into place.

CHAPTER SIX

STEP
6 # Maintain Loving Connections

W hen I was embattled in my own fight with food, I kept hearing how "social support" was critical to losing weight. At first, I was reluctant to invite help into this area of my life—it felt like being monitored by the food police—someone watching your every move to make sure you stick to your diet. I knew that would never work for me.

Actually, social support is the opposite of what I imagined. It's having your family, friends, and other trusted people help you lose weight. This is what Step 6 is all about.

Loving connections are extremely important if you want to make changes in your life. A few examples: Your spouse can participate in making healthy meals for you or buoy you up when the scale hasn't budged. Friends can share the latest and greatest tip, an encouraging word, a new exercise technique, or a healthy recipe. A co-worker can talk you through the urge to inhale the doughnuts in the break room, maybe getting you to go for a walk instead. A supportive dieting buddy can rejoice with you as another five pounds are shed. Someone else in your life might make a great accountability partner when the thought of skipping that walk or taking a bite of unhealthy food can be tempting.

In our go-it-alone world, it's tough to seek help for something as personal as your addictions. But the truth is, it's not just about food; it's about your life. And that life can be shattered by weight problems. More than two-thirds of us are now so heavy that health risks and full-fledged conditions are piling up. It's a health time bomb with the potential to explode over the next three decades into thousands of additional cases of heart disease, cancer, diabetes, arthritis, and more. Diabetes is a powerful example of this dangerous trend. The Centers for Disease Control (CDC) estimate that by the year 2050 as many as 1 in 3 U.S. adults could have type 2 diabetes (today 1 in 10 adults are afflicted). These and other alarming statistics show how critical it is for us to improve our lifestyle choices when it comes to eating and physical activity.

So don't be afraid to ask for the loving help you need. Realizing that others are cheering you on (and also keeping you accountable) gives you the extra motivation to stay the course.

Find a *Just 10* Buddy

The best support comes from family and friends, according to a *Journal of Consulting and Clinical Psychology* study that compared dieters grouped with supportive strangers to those who received encouragement from three friends or family members. Researchers found that 95 percent of participants in the friends-and-family group stuck with their weight-loss program and 66 percent were able to maintain their entire weight loss for 10 months. Only 24 percent of participants who entered the program without knowing the people in their support group kept the pounds off. We're all connected, so use those connections to achieve your *Just 10* goals.

I recommend that you find someone to do the *Just 10* program with you. My *Just 10* buddy is my brother Scott, who has lost 100 pounds on this program. I stay accountable to him, and he does to me. We share what we weigh, what we eat, our struggles, and our triumphs. To share all that was a jolt at first, like getting a shock from an improperly grounded light fixture. But we got past the shock, and it worked for us. I also have a workout buddy—Bryant. He helps me stay on top of my exercise program; and when I get off-track, I've given him permission to call me on it. In our work at Change Institute, where we coach people on losing weight, we encourage them to get connected with local support, because those who diet and exercise together also get slim together.

Ideally, your buddy (or buddies) should have the same goals as you do. That way, whenever temptation strikes (and it will—old habits die hard), you have each other to lean on for support. Friends might try to dissuade you from exercising in favor of some other activity, but support-group buddies encourage your desire to live lighter and better and change old patterns.

You've got to "hang" with like-minded people. There might be consequences if you don't. Landmark research published in 2007 in the *New England Journal of Medicine* reported that if a friend gains weight, your chances of mimicking her rise by 57 percent—even if she lives across the country.

In a sense, weight gain is contagious. But it's not that an actual bug is being passed from person to person. Rather, it's a more subtle transmission of behaviors. Maybe you and your husband like to eat out a lot. Or perhaps at work you eat cake at every celebration of co-workers' birthdays. Or you socialize a lot with friends whose favorite activity is eating. It's like the old saying "If you hang out at the barbershop long enough, you're gonna get a haircut."

Luckily this sort of peer pressure also works in a positive direction. The same research I mentioned above reported some good news, too. If you hang out with thin, fit people, you tend to be thinner and in better health. Dropping pounds is contagious; this is why it's important to surround yourself with friends who are as determined as you to make the numbers on the scale go down.

To lose weight, you can't—you mustn't—go it alone. Sure, your instinct will be to try to do this on your own, but you must resist. Successful weight loss depends on the help, love, and support of a hand-selected group of people. Being around like-minded people is encouraging and uplifting. When you're buoyed up and in a positive emotional state, it's easier to love yourself. So plug into inspiring, positive, loving people.

Make a list of those who might support you in your *Just 10* efforts. Ask yourself the following:

- **Is this person loving and supportive?** Be realistic and honest about personality traits. Don't expect Cousin Bonnie, for instance, to be anything other than who she is. If being loving and supportive aren't traits she has demonstrated in the past, cross her off the list.

- **Will he or she jump in to help you out of the weeds?** If your mom has been cruel and nags you about your extra pounds, rule her out as a support-group candidate. Find someone less emotionally invested. You need someone who will help, not condemn; push, not shame. Also, if you've started and stopped diet or exercise plans with your friend Heather in the past, don't turn to her this time. Seek out those who will have a fresh outlook.

- **Will this person hold you to your agreements?** You want people who aren't going to cave in if you do. You want people who will hold you accountable, but in a loving way.

- **Will this person be a good role model?** If it's Aunt Barbara, she may want to share her success. Ask about her diet or exercise habits, or if she would be willing to coach you or be a point person to whom you can report your progress. You don't need an Olympic or professional athlete to help you, just someone with good, consistent health and fitness habits.

Make sure your buddy understands what you're going through and that you need help. Then don't be afraid to lean on your buddy when you need to. He or she can get you through the tough days, and you can do the same in return.

You just never know when someone is going to offer just the right word of encouragement at just the right time. Not long ago,

I was in Seattle worshipping with my friends Reverend Michael Innersole and Reverend Kathianne Lewis at the Center for Spiritual Living. Reverend Kathianne asked me, "How good can you get?"

At first, I didn't understand what she meant. Then I got it: She was asking me, "How much good in your life can you stand?"

Later that evening, as a big storm moved in the area and rain pounded the windows with fury, her question hit me. "How good can you get?" Tears rolled down my cheeks as I thought about how good my life has become—how much healing has occurred and how much health has replaced the worry and garbage I lived with more than a decade ago. So much of the change came from the love I let others give me. I would not be writing these words or helping others without that support.

So let me ask you: How good can *you* get? How about all the way to great?

Strength in Numbers

You may not think you're the support-group type, but you might be surprised. Support groups typically have people with goals and experiences similar to yours. So many problems are so widely shared. You'll recognize your own problems in what other people are experiencing, and you might just find community in our go-it-alone culture. You'll also get a chance to hear about other people's successes. This can be very inspiring when friends can gather and speak freely in front of one another.

Support groups provide not only encouragement, but also mentoring, problem solving, and coaching. People who have a support group—of family or friends or an organized meeting—are more successful with long-term weight loss. I mentioned a research study earlier in the chapter, but the benefits of support are worth repeating and there is plenty of research to corroborate those benefits. In another study, men and women who participated in a structured weight-loss program that included weekly group support lost more weight and did a better job of keeping it off for two years than did people who lacked group support.

There are more than 500,000 support groups in the United States (that's a conservative estimate), serving upward of 20 million people. This figure includes branches and chapters of national organizations, as well as strictly local, independent groups.

Support groups exist in a variety of forms. Some are highly structured, others are informal. Some groups meet on a regular basis—once a week, once a month—in public places, or irregularly in the homes of members whenever schedules can be accommodated. There are even online support groups. Some work closely with health and psychology professionals, others don't. If you get involved in a support group for weight management, you'll feel less isolated knowing others share similar problems. You can also exchange ideas and effective ways to cope with problems and gain a new sense of control over your life.

If you initially attempted to lose weight on your own, then try one of these support options.

Check out existing groups such as GreySheeters Anonymous (GSA) or Overeaters Anonymous (OA), but be aware that meetings vary greatly. One meeting can be a winner and then the next several may be real duds. Give each group a couple chances before ruling it out. Use the following litmus test: if you find a particular meeting to be a room full of obese people who have been getting together largely unchanged and still overweight, check out another meeting. Seriously. I've been to these types of gatherings, as 12-step meetings are part of my own recovery support. I have walked into bum meetings in Chicago, Los Angeles, and every other part of the country only to find a terrific one in another part of whatever town I'm in. Misery loves company and 12-step support is only as healthy as the people in the group. So keep this in mind when giving 12-step or any kind of support a go. Simply try to see if it resonates with you after a fair length of time.

There are other support options out there. Your nearby gym is probably filled with people who are making similar lifestyle changes, and many of them offer structured support for members. I'm a member of a couple of gyms, and this makes my health-central circle a vibrant and accessible part of my daily life.

Online forums are another option. Several well-designed websites provide one-on-one consultations with nutritionists, fitness experts, and therapists, as well as online support groups where you can share with others who will understand and be eager to help.

To find support groups in your community, check the following: community bulletin board sections of your local newspaper or cable TV provider, your family doctor, local hospitals, social service agencies, churches, and online. You'll find a lot of information about these and other avenues of support at my online resource center at *Just10Diet.com.*

Start Your Own Support Group

If you can't find a support group but recognize its value, consider starting your own. Here are some suggestions to help you get started:

- **Turn to friends and family for a support group.** Some of them may welcome the suggestion, particularly if they want to lose weight, too. Have a rational discussion about the benefits of support and back it up with the study data I've provided in this book. Be specific about what kind of support you need: socializing activities that don't focus solely on food. Present fun, healthy activities that promote physical fitness but that aren't intimidating, like Frisbee golf or hula hooping. Explain that they don't have to upend their own lives, but they should at least support your *Just 10* plan. Communicate very clearly how important this is for you and how important your goals are. Let them know that you need their support, love, and encouragement through actions, not just words.

- **Start a *Just 10* group at work.** In many places, employees are banding together to lose weight, sometimes at the urging of bosses who are worried about health insurance costs, the effects of obesity on workplace productivity, and the emotional and physical well-being of their teams.

They're starting contests à la the reality show *The Biggest Loser* or just sharing fresh, raw veggies or fruit during break instead of a box of cookies.

Though some employees or employers might find the trend too intrusive, others welcome on-the-job dieting as a weight-control tool. Look, the truth is that we as a nation are getting reckless with the food problem. The competitive nature of so many business environments—which has probably helped us get into our obesity predicament—can, in fact, become a motivating place to do better.

If you decide to start a *Just 10* group at work, make sure it's okay with your employer. If not, find somewhere outside of your workplace to start your group.

- **Decide the parameters of your group.** Where and when will you meet? How often will you meet? How long will the meeting last? Will you facilitate it, have rotating leaders, or let it be more free-form? You can get a *Just 10* group guide with more ideas online at *Just10Diet.com*.

- **Schedule weekly weigh-ins (or not).** Decide as a group if you want to do weekly weigh-ins. It's up to you! I actually like to have my Change Institute clients weigh in daily just to stay in touch with their numbers—which never lie. The simple act of knowing you'll be weighing yourself can be an incentive to eat well. Others might feel uncomfortable doing group weigh-ins, but be open to making the suggestion, modifying it to suit everyone's privacy needs, and then honoring the consensus.

- **Have an agenda for your meetings.** Maybe each week is devoted to studying one of the steps. Encourage everyone to share *Just 10* strategies that work for them. Give everyone a chance to speak up. Listen and avoid cross-talk. Conclude with inspiration, such as a reading or an affirmation.

You might also have the group do moving meditation for some of your meetings. Or you can ask members to donate a few bucks to a rewards fund. Use the money to provide small prizes such as a gift certificate to a health-food store or donation to a deserving group or cause. At every session, treat one member who has been particularly successful.

Whether your group consists of friends, family, co-workers, or all of the above, the most important part is to have like-minded people who all share the same objective.

Not too long ago, I helped several women start a *Just 10* group at work, in connection with *The Dr. OZ Show*. These women—Lisa, Doree, Roberta, and Loraine—had worked together for years at a salon. They lived, laughed, loved, ate, and got heavy together. They e-mailed *The Dr. OZ Show*, asking for help. Dr. Oz asked me to go on a secret mission and do a "Craving Intervention" because they were having such a hard time getting started when their salon was a literal buffet. There was food everywhere: chocolates, pretzels, candies, caramels, doughnuts, bagels, and cookies. You name it, it was there and competing for these ladies' attention.

We made several changes immediately. The first was a tool I call "Extinction," which is a fancy way of saying we got rid of all the temptations. You can't eat what's not there. The Salon Ladies (my name for the group) made a commitment that the goodies would go the way of the dodo bird.

I also shared a tool with The Salon Ladies called "Rub It In," which is a form of positive reinforcement. It involves complimenting a person on the progress they've made but with a twist. For example, Lisa might say to Loraine: "Loraine, I am so proud of the effort you're making, and the commitment you're showing to be a healthier woman and a role model for your children. You are doing great!" I'd then ask Loraine to Rub It In. To rub in a compliment, you literally reach out and "catch" the words in the air with your hands, place your hands over your heart (or the heart of the person you're complimenting), and rub in the loving compliment. I do this with clients all the time. We take the words and accept them as love—and rub it in.

Rub It In might seem a little offbeat or hokey, but so often we get a compliment, discount it, and toss it aside. If we don't learn how to accept compliments, we are losing out on love and encouragement. Catching the compliment and rubbing it in grabs it, honors it, and touches your heart. Trust me, it's powerful and you'll like it. The Salon Ladies loved this tool and they still use it as part of living healthier, lighter, and better.

If you're struggling with weight and food issues, don't keep the problems to yourself and don't run from them. Circle the wagons. Get in a support group. We humans are communal beings. We thrive when we work together and share our experiences and our abilities. To enhance the quality of your life, turn to the people whom you love and trust, and turn to people who have learned to deal with similar problems. Ask for support, accept support, and count your blessings, because you will lose weight and your life will improve.

Try My Change Institute

Several years ago, I founded Change Institute because I knew that the two leading causes of death in America (smoking and obesity) are preventable, and I had to do something. My team and I began to work with clients on a structured food and weight-loss program that would help them change what they eat, how they eat, and why they eat. As part of Change Institute, we provide a free virtual community center, a place to gather and discuss the importance of embracing change.

An online community can be effective for many people, particularly in the beginning stages of change when you might be too timid to venture into a conventional support group. One of my first Change Institute clients was Cathy. She asked me to intervene with her son, but it turned out Cathy needed as much help as her son did. At age 44 and 5 foot 4, she was dying from obesity. Her blood pressure was 190/110, her cholesterol was 315, and she weighed 380 pounds. She also suffered from severe sleep apnea, a potentially life-threatening condition.

Cathy hadn't always been overweight, but over the course of seven years, she gained a substantial amount after some trying times raising her kids. Her daughter was date-raped, and her son became an alcoholic and drug addict. In response to these heart-breaking events, Cathy regularly binged on food to numb out, and soon she became dangerously heavy.

Desperate, she tried just about every diet known to mankind. In 2005, she had Lap-Band surgery but told only her husband about it and refused the group support offered afterward. She wanted to prove that she could "do it herself." The surgery wasn't the miracle she'd expected; Cathy continued to overeat. As I hear time and time again, she "ate through the band."

She ballooned in size. Everyday tasks, such as tying her shoes or getting behind the wheel of a car, were extremely difficult. "I got so fat that I had to get a bigger car. That was when I knew, I just knew, I was going to die because of my food problem," she cried. It got to a point when even lying down was hard and sleep became nearly impossible. She knew she had to try again. She had to do something.

I worked with her on the 10 steps. Hardest of all was this step, Step 6—maintaining a loving connection to others. Cathy was always worried about what other people thought of her and felt too self-conscious and ashamed to attend group meetings. I suggested she try an online support group through Change Institute, where she could be anonymous but still receive the encouragement she needed. Cathy was game.

Over the next two years, Cathy lost 190 pounds. Food no longer ruled her life, and she learned how to live with her feelings and handle stresses in a healthy, life-affirming way. She credited online support with keeping her accountable and helping her to avoid roadblocks. People noticed her weight loss and asked her about her diet. Some suggested that Cathy start and lead a support group. She hesitated at first because she didn't feel comfortable approaching people about their weight. But she knew the importance of sur-rounding yourself with people who want you to achieve your goals. Eventually, she formed a group at church, starting with just two friends. Their effort was contagious. Today, there are more than 30 people in the group. Cathy says, "There is absolutely no charge. It's free. We're just a group of people helping each other. I turned the thing I thought was going to kill me into a blessing."

Wow! I love that.

Consider Professional Support

A lot of people may benefit from professional support, such as a dietician, nutritionist, or therapist. Dieticians and nutritionists can help you with meal planning; a therapist can counsel you on your eating habits and issues with food. Let's examine both.

Nutritional Counseling

Dieticians and nutritionists have the training to deliver accurate, personalized nutrition advice. You might want to add one to your support team. Here are some things to consider.

What motivates you? Are you the type of person who needs detailed menus and daily "nutrition policing"? If so, you should choose a nutritionist whose counseling style meets those needs. If you only need motivation to follow your diet, then a person who pushes biweekly meetings and weigh-ins at the office is not right for you. If you're a socially oriented learner who likes discussing your experiences with others, then be sure to ask about group counseling and support groups. While most nutritionists can accommodate a variety of client styles, it is important to have a good grasp of the amount of motivation, supervision, and follow-up you will need to achieve your goals before you set your first appointment.

Discuss your *Just 10* goals. Put your thoughts, progress, and struggles down on paper in your journal or your *Just 10 Workbook*. Although a nutritionist can help you define problem areas in your diet through a variety of techniques (interviews, questionnaires, diet journaling, and perhaps computer diet analysis), it's still up to you to clarify that you're focused on losing the first 10 pounds, and you're using specific steps to help you. Talk to the nutritionist about

Just 10 and explain that you need his or her support in following through.

To find a dietician or nutritionist:

- Get referrals from your physician or local hospital.

- Request a list of private practice professionals from your state Department of Public Health.

- Contact your local chapter of the American Dietetic Association (*www.eatright.org*) or American Society for Clinical Nutrition (*www.nutrition.org*).

- Try word of mouth. Friends can often be a good source of recommendations. Put this as your Facebook update: "Doing *Just 10 Lbs*. Who wants to join me? Who knows of a great nutritionist?"

Mental-Health Counseling

Time and again, I hear, "I'm crazy when it comes to food." You're not likely crazy, but you likely do some crazy things around food. Feelings of isolation and depression frequently go hand in hand with an out-of-control food story. I understand and have been through it myself and with many clients. Remember this, too: Food, just like many drugs, affects your brain. It tweaks your brain and changes how you feel.

The key here is to not run to a mental-health counselor such as a psychiatrist to throw a pill at the problem. I had a psychiatrist who prescribed Xanax for me for nearly a decade. I was anxious over my litany of issues, and her diagnosis always treated my symptoms. "I sweat, and I'm extremely anxious," I told her. She kept me on the pills for years.

A good mental-health counselor or therapist can help you work through some deeper issues regarding your food and eating behavior. Any therapist you select should be licensed by the state. Find out their academic and professional credentials. Some have masters degrees in social work or counseling, some have Ph.D.'s in psychology, and some are medical doctors.

When considering a counselor, ask about their experience: how long they have been in practice, what kind of training do they have, whether or not they have a specialty, if they are affiliated with an academic institution, and so on. Find out whether the therapist has ever dealt with your particular problem before. If so, how often? If the therapist doesn't have the expertise you need, he should be willing to refer you to a therapist better able to handle the issues you're facing.

Some very good counselors might not even be credentialed as professionals, but they might be helpful because they struggled with the same food issues themselves. These "lay counselors" can be very helpful, particularly as role models. You can learn from them and adopt some of their success strategies as your own.

There should be a certain connection or chemistry between you and the therapist. So how do you know? I believe every last one of us has a small, still voice inside our head that acts as a barometer of what is right and good. Seek out that voice, inside you now. If you're not sure the counselor is someone you can work with, don't waste time trying. Move on to someone else. Sometimes you have to look around a little before you find the right person.

If money is an issue, certain faith-based programs are often willing to serve people without insurance or financial resources. People who work in these programs share a deep commitment to serve for little or no money. Understand that faith-based providers usually make their general religious tenets known from the beginning and use the language and teachings of religion to reach clients, instead of relying on clinical language alone. If this doesn't sit well with you, then a secular program may be better. But for many people, if you have no insurance, no money, no family support, and perhaps even no job, this is an alternative worth looking into. Be open to hearing their message, and take what you can from it. Many churches have support groups modeled after Weigh Down and Celebrate Recovery, which are two groups you can search for online to find meetings and support near you.

Losing just 10 pounds is not something that happens in a vacuum. It must be accomplished through loving relationships with not only the self, but with others. The sixth step to loving yourself and weighing what you want entails making sure that you maintain close supportive relationships with people who care about you and want to see you reach your goals. Just keep reminding yourself that you're worth it, and hang in there.

Take 10

1. Support breaks down feelings of isolation. In the support group, in particular, you discover the commonality of your experiences and feelings and learn from and find hope in each other's struggles and triumphs.

2. As you seek support, clarify in your own mind why you would like to join a group. To gather information? Get emotional support? Learn from others how to deal with weight management? More than likely it's some combination of reasons.

3. Decide whether you prefer the anonymity of a larger group or the increased intimacy of a smaller one, such as a group you might form with your family and friends.

4. Some groups are led by a therapist or other professional. Others are peer-led. Decide which you prefer.

5. Determine whether you prefer members to be the same age or a range of ages. Would you feel comfortable around only the same gender or is a co-ed group okay?

6. Consider how membership fits into your lifestyle by looking at such things as the frequency and length of meetings, and time of day they're held.

7. Some support or therapy groups might charge a fee. Check to see if your insurance covers it.

8. Within a support group, you may find a weight-loss buddy you can work with outside the group for extra support and encouragement.

9. If you join a support group and lose weight, your success can rub off on your spouse or partner. A study from the University of Connecticut says that couples not only tend to gain weight together, they can also lose it as a pair, even if only one of them is enrolled in a formal program.

10. The first support group you join may not be the perfect one for you. Keep looking, and you will come closer to finding what you are looking for.

JUST 10 MYTH BUSTER
WE CAN CHANGE ON OUR OWN

If we could change on our own, we'd do it in a heart-beat. After all, who wants to live a life that has spun out of control? Who wants to be super-sized? Who wants to feel uncomfortable, in a body that hurts? Who wants to be drunk or strung out on drugs all the time? Who wants to lie awake at night, terrified of one thing or another? Who wants to be stressed out, scared, or uncertain about what's next?

Let's look at the odds. People rarely, if ever, change entirely on their own. Allow me to use myself as an example again. I had been smoking since 1981, drinking since 1982, doing cocaine and other drugs since 1984, and eating compulsively the entire time. By the time I attended my first 12-step meeting for my addiction problems back in 1991, I had a solid decade of disordered behavior behind me. I went to meetings, tail tucked between my legs, ashamed to be there. I attended meetings like this off and on for two years. I even celebrated an uninterrupted year of sobriety in the group. The only trouble was, I was living a lie. I went to meetings off and on yet never spoke to another soul. I kept my head down while expecting that some kind of 12-step osmosis would occur just from showing up on occasion. I was worn down, worn out, and brittle.

I chose to leave my dream job as a TV weather anchor because it was interfering with my addictions. My friends were shocked at my decision to walk away. My agent was ticked off. I switched careers anyway.

I was in such deep denial about my addiction that I actually went into the food-and-beverage business. Can you believe it—food and alcohol, of all things! I was so successful at it that I opened a dance club in short order, then a lounge.

In reality, my new careers were yet another excuse to stay in sickness with impunity.

Looking back over that period in my life, it became clear to me that if someone had stepped in and talked to me and had done some form of intervention earlier, I would have gotten help immediately. I would have said yes, and I would have stopped using all sorts of drugs to numb out. But instead, I thought I had it under control, that I would be able to quit on my own. "I'll quit tomorrow," I would say to myself—but tomorrow didn't come until much later.

A great deal had to happen before I could change. You would think that blacking out almost every day from alcohol or throwing up digested food into the toilet would do that, but in my case it did not. And so it went. I lied and deflected blame, and the hole I dug for myself got deeper and deeper. Denial—first of drinking, then of the self—stretched to include more and more bits of reality; and after a while, I could not see the truth, could not see who I was or what I needed. If I could have stopped, I would have. I wanted to eat, snort, drink, smoke, and consume to get outside of what and how I was feeling.

Quitting was simply not possible without help—even in the face of severe consequences. When a friend insisted I get help without negotiation or delay, I took the next step, which involved rehab, therapy, and consistent group support. And for me, that's how change began.

CHAPTER SEVEN

STEP 7

Eliminate Excuses

Although it wasn't obvious to me when I was struggling with food and drugs, I was hiding behind a lot of excuses. I'd tell myself things like, *I need this stuff to cope,* or *I'm too fat to exercise.* Then I would justify a binge by saying to myself, *Just this once, and I'll make changes on Monday,* or *I'll eat a few slices of birthday cake because I don't want to offend the birthday boy.* How many similar excuses have you used when trying to justify your own behavior?

I was always so good at rationalizing my bad habits. I had excuses at the ready for every circumstance. I just wanted to hang on to my bad habits for dear life. What I hadn't realized was that they were costing me my dear life!

I knew eventually I wouldn't be able to hide behind excuses anymore. Excuses had to be replaced with action, however imperfect or inadequate. I had to give up eating and drinking whatever I wanted and as much as I wanted. I could no longer obey that siren voice urging me to eat food full of fat and sugar. I had to replace undisciplined eating with deliberate eating, and I had to stop using food and drink recreationally. Giving up the excuses helped me get on the path to change.

Making excuses is a bad habit that anyone can slip into. I've done it, you've done it, and now it's time to get past it. This is what Step 7 is all about.

The Cupcake Story

This is a story to illustrate how our crafty minds work. Let's say I'm diet-ing to lose weight. I crave a cupcake but feel torn between the desire for the cupcake and the need to stay on my diet. I've got those two con-flicting thoughts in my head at the same time. Eat the cupcake; don't eat the cupcake. This typically creates a feeling of uncomfortable ten-sion. Psychologists call this conflict "cognitive dissonance." It's based on the idea that we can experience psychological distress when we have beliefs or attitudes that are incongruous or opposites.

For instance, I like cupcakes, but I'm also trying to lose weight. These two thoughts are incompatible: if I eat the cupcake, then I may gain weight, and if I really want to lose weight then I cannot eat the cupcake. These are referred to as "dissonant" ideas.

The basic premise of cognitive dissonance is that humans don't like to have dissonant ideas (or cognitions). They make us feel uncomfort-able and conflicted. As a result, we try to do away with the dissonance.

For example, I might ignore or eliminate the conflicting thought. I might pretend that cupcakes aren't bad for me, that I can have my cupcake and eat it, too. Ignoring the conflicting thought allows me to do things I might otherwise view as wrong, inappro-priate, or unhealthy.

Second, I might alter the importance of certain cognitions. I might decide that I can't do without cupcakes or that losing weight isn't as important as eating the cupcakes. That way, I lessen the uncomfortable feeling of dissonance so that I don't feel so bad about eating cupcakes.

Third, I might create a bunch of new ideas. For instance, I could rationalize eating the cupcake because "I exercise three times a week," or "I need some carbs," or "I had a small dinner," or "I don't want to offend the person who baked the cupcakes," and so on. The more cognitions—excuses—I come up with, the more justified I feel to eat the cupcake. The multiple cognitions that say eating the cupcake is okay overwhelm the one cognition that says eating the cupcake would be bad for me.

Finally, I might deal with cognitive dissonance by avoiding it. If I'm presented with information that is dissonant from what I already know, the easiest way to deal with this new information is to ignore it, refuse to accept it, or simply postpone acknowledging it. Suppose a new study comes out that says cupcakes are more fattening than scientists originally thought. I'd eat my cupcakes now and deal with that pesky study later.

In each case, to release the tension, I'm coming up with a bunch of clever excuses to eat the cupcake. The excuses give me a reason to say, "Go ahead . . . eat the cupcake." The problem is, though, that if you keep making excuses, you won't lose weight.

The solution is to know your typical excuses, how you justify your behavior, and how to work around excuses and behaviors so that you reach your *Just 10* goal. Step 7 will help.

What's Your Excuse?

We're all guilty of coming up with excuses about why we can't possibly change what we eat, or leave our comfy sofa and do some exercise. This isn't right or wrong; this is just human nature.

The trick is to dig deep and look rationally at your typical excuses. What are your excuses? Make a list of them. Seriously. Do it, before I show up at your home and put a pen in your hand.

I have them still, and now they're usually around travel. When I'm on the road for the fourth day and I'm tired and feeling run down and worn out, they'll creep in . . . just one . . . no, just five . . . "Drink me!!!" . . . "Eat me!!!" . . . You know the voices.

Your excuses are not helping you lose weight, so let's counter them with positive strategies. To help you get started, take a look at the excuses my client Joanna listed in her journal after starting my program. She has used all of these to justify going off her diet:

- It's the Fourth of July.

- My family is in town.

- It's a potluck dinner.

- It's Friday.

- It's Wednesday.

- It's my birthday.

- It's payday.

- We're in love.

- It's a full moon!

- It's her birthday.

- It's his birthday.

- The ocean is blue.

- We're on vacation.

- I'm tired.

- I got a raise.

- I got a huge contract.

- I had a great day.

- I had a bad day.

Let's take one of Joanna's excuses as an example: I got a huge contract. In the past, she'd go out and celebrate with a huge meal. That's a bad idea for Joanna if she's trying to lose weight, because it's easy to eat several hundred calories without thinking. Then there's the post-meal guilt. Joanna feels so bad afterward, that going off her diet starts a spiral of overeating and weight gain, and she beats herself up every time.

The strategies we identified included sticking with her *Just 10* commitment. She agreed to:

- Plan and commit to what she'd eat prior to going out.

- Hone her dining-out strategies to choose healthier, more *Just 10*–friendly foods.

- Eat smaller portions. Joanna eventually learned that she didn't have to eat a big meal to be sociable or to celebrate.

- Enjoy some nonfood activities to celebrate, such as buying concert tickets or new clothes. Get a manicure, pedicure, or massage. Light some candles and have special time with her husband. Once the new nonfood choices became associated with achievement and joy, they stuck and became her new norm. Joanna learned to reward herself with healthier choices.

So the key is this: figure out the excuses you use to justify your behavior. What usually stops you from eating well or exercising? Maybe you always found reasons to avoid the gym after work. Write them down. Come up with an alternate activity that seems feasible, like walking before breakfast. If it rains (weather is always a good excuse to justify behavior), perhaps you'll do yoga in your living room with a DVD or using one of our online workouts at *Just10Diet.com*.

Without concrete plans, it's difficult to work toward your goals.

Before you make excuses, ask yourself, *What will this do for me?* Often we overlook the consequences of our behavior. The "I'll cross that bridge when I get there" mentality can be devastating. Become proactive and work to avoid the bridge altogether. Don't wait for your bad choices to exact their cost. Start making healthy decisions now.

We just looked at Joanna's excuses. Now let's look at some other common excuses, plus strategies to use if you're dealing with some of the same issues. Knowing your excuses and strategizing around them are powerful ways to lose just 10 pounds (and more!).

Common Excuses

What I want to do is unravel the eight most common excuses that I hear from people we coach. Let's start with the ace of spades, the "I'm-too-busy" card. That one gets a lot of play.

1. I don't have time to get in shape.

The time problem is magnified for many people by their choice of priorities. And, unfortunately for many, fitness doesn't rank. This is especially true for businesspeople, who put their jobs before everything, and for moms, who often prioritize the needs of their family above their own. "As I'm walking on the treadmill, I'm thinking of all the other things I should be doing," one of my clients told me. Or as a busy mom confided, "I have to get up at 6 A.M. for work. I have to do the laundry. I've got to get the kids off to school. I don't always have time to prepare good meals."

The fix lies in a simple adjustment in perspective and daily organization. What we have to realize is that if we're not fit and healthy, we won't be able to fulfill the rest of our obligations as effectively. If we're not modeling life-affirming behaviors for our kids, they will become part of the generation that's predicted to die before their parents from obesity-related diseases. In my own work, I try to get my clients on board with this idea: you don't have time *not* to exercise and eat healthy.

It's all about liking yourself enough to take care of yourself. Wouldn't you rather your family, friends, and associates see what a rock star you are? Wouldn't you rather your kids see how strong, fit, capable, and self-respecting and self-loving you are? After all, it is you they learn from and mimic. Want to be the best mom or dad you can be for your kids? Start exercising now. You can even turn fitness into family fun and include the kids.

Simply reorganize the day and incorporate healthy activities into it. Map out your weekly schedule, writing in all the key appointments, errands, and kids' activities, and you'll see where your time goes each week. Then you can identify open slots for food preparation, unrushed meals, and exercise.

If you're pressed for food preparation time, stock up on ready-made meals (preferably with fewer than 400 calories and 20 grams of fat), but bump up the nutritional content by adding a large bowl of prewashed and ready-to-eat salad greens and a handful of cherry tomatoes.

If you think about it and are honest with yourself, this isn't a time-management problem. It's a self-management problem. If you have time to watch a couple hours of TV every day, you have time to prepare healthy meals or do a workout. It was a great relief when I discovered I could bike for 45 minutes on a recumbent bike and have a good cardiovascular workout all the while catching up on my reading and TV shows.

Some other time vacuums: if you have time to go to happy hour after work, you have time to work out. If you have time to be on Facebook, Twitter, and YouTube, you have time to do healthy activities.

Contrary to popular belief, or popular excuses, eating healthy foods or exercising isn't more time consuming than the other activities I've mentioned. Like anything else, it just takes knowledge and practice. Remember, following a healthful lifestyle doesn't require an all-or-nothing approach; every positive change helps. And your body will thank you in the long run. So here's to positive change and very long runs!

2. I can't give up going out to eat.

Who says you have to?

Following a few simple guidelines will help you lose weight without turning into a hermit.

- **Use your eyes and newfound common sense.** If the order starts with "Supersize number four" you're still on the wrong track. Gather information by getting to know and commit to your food plan. Go online and check the restaurant's menu beforehand. I even encourage my clients to decide what they're going to order before they get to the restaurant, where the sights and smells can blow even the best of intentions.

- **Be first.** Order before anyone else to avoid letting others' choices influence you.

- **Choose alcoholic drinks carefully.** Booze is packed with calories and can make or break a diet. It also lowers your inhibitions and sets the stage for overeating. How many times has your no-dessert plan gone out the window after the second or third glass of wine? The best option is not to have any at all, or just a little like a single measure of liquor with a calorie-free mixer, a glass of wine, or light beer.

- **Go halvsies.** Ask the restaurants to use only half of the normal portion for high-fat ingredients such as cheese, oil, white sauce, or gravy. That way, you get the flavor without overdoing it.

- **Order extra veggies.** I love to order sides of healthily prepared greens and veggies of all kinds. They have become the cornerstone of my nutritional lifestyle, and they've helped my clients reshape their bodies. Just make simple changes at first, and eventually the new habits will replace the old. Whether the veggies are packed in a sandwich, are a side dish, or are part of a stir-fry, ask for an extra helping of these low-cal, high-fiber gems.

- **Share often.** Offer a taste of your dish to everyone at your table. The more they eat, the less there is for you. When it's time for dessert, I always ask myself: *Am I full? Have I had enough?* If I still want and/or need something else, I'll ask for a small bowl of fresh fruit.

- **Skip the high-calorie apps.** Have a nice, simple self-loving salad. Alternatively, ask for two appetizers and have one as your main course. Good appetizers include smoked salmon, prawn cocktail (without cocktail sauce), vegetable soup, tomato and mozzarella salad with balsamic vinegar, or a green salad.

- **Cut your meals in half.** Take the second half home in a doggie bag. Portions are often too large in restaurants these days.

- **Select grilled meat, poultry, or fish with salad.** These are all great choices for a main course.

- **Opt for a fresh fruit salad or sorbet over other desserts.** As a rule, avoid anything that's fried or made with loads of butter, cream, pastry, or cheese.

- **Get real.** This isn't your last (restaurant) supper. You'll go out to eat again—probably to the very same place—so you don't have to eat everything that sounds good this time.

3. I can't afford to eat healthfully.

I agree that in many cases healthy food is more expensive, and it's easy to pass up healthful choices because of cost concerns. Recently, a study came out, noting that a diet rich in phytonutrient-packed blueberries might reverse certain age-related declines and improve short-term memory. Preliminary results from Tufts University scientists show that people who ate a cup of the berries a day performed better on motor skill tests than a control group. A cup a day? Who are they kidding? My local grocery store charges $3 for a measly six-ounce container.

But the truth is you *can* find healthy food on the cheap. The myth that healthy food is more costly than FrankenFood is just that—a myth!

New York Times food writer Mark Bittman blew this myth out of the water with his eye-opening piece, "Is Junk Food Really Cheaper?" He showed that a dinner of roast chicken, vegetables, salad, and milk, which will feed four to six people, is cheaper than the far less nutritious FrankenFood meal they'd buy at McDonald's.

And yes, some healthy food can be costly. But we still need to eat it; let's just be smart about our choices and the costs attached to them. I love frozen berries—and they're often more cost effective than the fresh ones. Winter squash, peppers, peas, and carrots are in my freezer, too. They're a staple for me and for so many of my private coaching clients.

- **Enjoy some preserved foods.** Don't assume that fresh is always best; some preserved foods have even higher nutrient levels. Canned tomatoes, for example, are higher in lycopene than fresh tomatoes and are a more economical, nutritious, and eco-friendly choice than off-season tomatoes, picked green and shipped across the country. I have rarely met a canned tomato I didn't like—and my cupboard is always stocked with stewed tomatoes.

- **Eat more plant-based foods.** Americans tend to plan their menus around the most expensive (and highest in saturated fat) item: meat. Health experts suggest that your plate should be split in thirds. Two-thirds should be plant foods (fruits, vegetables, whole grains, legumes, seeds, nuts) with less than one-third of animal protein. I concur. This fraction might astonish you—but I want you to wrap your head and heart around it. 2/3 + 1/3 = 3/3. It's a great way to visualize your plate and what you should be eating to get and stay healthy.

- **Avoid wasting food.** While it's not a healthy habit to clean your plate when you're not hungry, people waste far too much food. An estimated 40 to 50 percent of food that is harvested in the United States never gets eaten. That number amazes me, and my heart hurts as I know so many people in this country (and in other parts of the world, as well) go to sleep hungry. Bottom line: cut down on portion size and save your leftovers for lunch the next day. This will make your bottom and your bottom line happy.

- **Brown bag it.** Instead of spending your dining dollars on fast-food runs or vending machine snacks, pack a healthy lunch using dinner leftovers or wholesome sandwiches, fruits, and vegetables. I love a healthy whole-wheat wrap packed with veggies, mustard, and some protein or hummus.

- **Cut out low-nutrient foods.** If your food dollars are on a diet, then so should your pantry be. Who needs low-nutrient junk foods that add little more than calories, sodium, fat, and chemicals to your diet? Instead, shop for nutrient-rich whole foods like yogurt, fruits, grains, nuts, and veggies.

- **Make shopping lists.** This helps prevent impulse buys and expensive, calorie-packed biscuits, cakes, chips, and booze.

- **Buy fruits and vegetables in season from a local market.** Not only are they often cheaper in your local market, but buying there is also a great way to connect with your community. I've never met a farmer's market I didn't like. Try one soon, and see how you can integrate it into your own eating lifestyle.

4. I don't want to give up my favorite foods.

You might need to eat fewer of them, or smaller portions, but dieting doesn't mean ditching your faves. Write in your journal or your *Just 10 Workbook* exactly how many snacks you eat a day. You'll probably be surprised by the amount.

Then allow yourself a 100- to 200-calorie treat every day. The challenge here is this: snack on foods that don't trigger you. If your snack leads to a binge, take that food off your food plan for the time being.

The strategy is to eat a little bit of what you love when you get the urge. Banning desired foods from your diet can make you crave them more. So for many dieters, it helps to eat a little of your favorite foods during the week. You could even substitute a lower-calorie version of your favorite treat. If you love chocolate, for example, have some reduced-calorie hot chocolate.

There is room for moderation, but a lot of this stuff may represent trigger foods for you. As a recovering alcoholic and binge eater, I don't drink alcohol or eat processed foods anymore, period. So if you have some of those items that just don't work for you, abstain from them and see how you feel. Or try the following techniques:

One is called "thought-stopping." Many bad habits are triggered by unhelpful thoughts and ruminations. The longer such thoughts hang around in your head, the more they make themselves at home and sabotage your actions.

The minute a negative thought (*I want to eat the whole cake*) arises, say to yourself either out loud or silently, "Stop it!" Then relax for a few seconds and switch to a more helpful thought, such as a slim you in a bathing suit. Some people are advised to wear a rubber band—or the *Just 10* bracelet mentioned in Chapter 1—on their wrist that they snap whenever the negative thought comes to mind. The objective is to stop destructive thoughts before they get out of control.

Another technique is to develop a competing response. One of the keys to eliminating a poor habit is to replace it with a better one—which is why competing responses are so powerful. A competing response is a behavior that is incompatible with the habit. If you feel like bingeing, for example, take a shower or go for a run. It's hard to eat a whole cake in the shower or while running. If you learn to do this more often, you'll eventually lose the urge to binge. By making the new habit incompatible with the old one, the bad one will naturally decrease in strength, since the two cannot coexist.

Or just simply go into relaxation mode. Deep breathing is a good way to ease the stress and anxiety that triggers destructive habits like bingeing. When you begin to feel overwhelmed or anxious, stop for a few minutes and take some slow deep breaths. This will calm you down, clear your mind of unnecessary clutter, and give you a better sense of control. Remember, having feelings of hunger are good. We're built for it. This kind of normal hunger will not kill and will not threaten your health. So love yourself with foods that feed all of you, not just your cravings or feelings. Take that love and hold it close to you.

5. I need food to deal with stress.

Stress is a fact of daily life, and many of us cope by medicating ourselves with food. If you're the type who gets stressed while at work or if you get that 2 P.M. snack attack at the office, plan ahead by leaving the vending-machine change at home and planting your office with body-honoring snacks. Break up your knee-jerk eating habit by taking a walk around the block or shutting your office door and taking a few minutes to breathe deeply and listen to relaxing music.

If you're the type who medicates with food outside the office, I have a better idea: engage in creative pursuits. Two of my favorite things in life are playing the piano and writing music. I've learned to channel stress and anxiety through these activities. If I do both, I can be content for hours and hours. They leave me feeling clear, calm, and fully connected to my authentic self.

If you've never discovered the simple pleasure of creativity, start by coming up with a list of creative activities that you enjoy so you can quickly turn to them when you feel stressed and close to a binge. If you currently have no hobbies, think back to when you were a kid. What kind of activities did you like to do? Paint? Take photographs? Write? What type of creative classes did you take in school? Write them down in your journal or your *Just 10 Workbook*.

Also, think about creative pursuits you've never explored, but have always wanted to. Have you always been fascinated by acting, singing, or playing an instrument? Do you love flipping through decorating magazines and gazing at beautifully designed rooms? Make a list of your passions, and then brainstorm how you might pursue them.

Finally, participate in them—and participate as often as you can, and especially when you feel troublesome emotions beginning to creep in. Sing. Paint. Write poetry. Play the guitar. Dance. Over time, you'll get used to expressing your feelings in positive ways without turning to food, and eating and living consciously will become a habit all its own.

6. I have a slow metabolism.

If I had a dollar for every time I hear someone claim they are overweight because of a slow metabolism, I'd be mighty rich! Metabolism refers to the amount of energy (calories) your body burns up in a day. Most people burn up calories at around the same rate. If you're overweight, you probably have a faster metabolism than someone who's slim. The heavier you are, the harder your body has to work to move around. This means you need more calories to keep your weight steady and so should find it easier to lose weight.

Repeated, or yo-yo, dieting doesn't slow down your metabolism permanently, either. In fact, you should be able to lose weight as effectively whether you are trying for the first time or are a seasoned dieter.

As for age, metabolism does slow as we age. For women there's a big drop with menopause. For other people, experts estimate that between ages 40 and 80, an average person's metabolism slows down by 25 to 30 percent.

There's a lot you can do to make sure your metabolism operates at peak efficiency, however. Here are some strategies:

- **Eat breakfast.** It's the most important thing you can do to burn calories faster. When experts from the University of Colorado Health Sciences Center surveyed about 3,000 men and women who had lost 130 pounds or more and had kept the weight off for at least a year, they found that breakfast was the one common denominator all the successful dieters shared. Your metabolism slows while you sleep, and the process of digesting food in the morning revs it up again. The sooner you eat after waking up, the better.

- **Tone your muscles.** Include some strength training as part of your moving meditation. The American College of Sports Medicine says that people can burn up to 200 calories with 30 minutes of strength training daily. It boosts muscle, which burns calories faster than either fat or untoned muscle.

- **Drink six to eight glasses of water daily.** Being dehydrated decreases your body's ability to burn calories by 2 percent each day, according to research from the University of Utah. I see a lot of people who don't get enough water without even realizing it. Your thirst mechanism often doesn't kick in until you're already dehydrated. Check your urine: If it's dark yellow instead of light yellow or clear, that's a sign that you're not drinking enough. I used to get most of my water through beer, vodka, and coffee. Now I get it through plain old water, herbal tea, and coffee. I drink six glasses of water a day, and add to the cistern with the tea and java.

- **Don't forget your daily practice.** When researchers from Oregon Health Sciences University checked in 18 months after overweight women had taken up relaxation techniques, they found that the women had each lost about 10 pounds without trying. One theory: since these women were less stressed, they weren't flooding their body with stress hormones, which are known to increase appetite and belly fat. Your daily practice will help make this happen.

7. My spouse/partner/kids won't eat healthy stuff.

No one wants the hassle of cooking separate meals, so make family dinners healthier without making a big deal about it—chances are everyone's health will also benefit. Go affirmative. Don't ask permission to give love in this way. Just do it.

- **Reduce the fat.** Use lower-fat products such as extra-lean meat and reduced-fat sausages, reduced-fat milk and part-skim cheeses. There are so many great-tasting, lower-calorie, and naturally low-fat foods, no one will know the difference.

- **Get sneaky.** Sneak some extra veggies into chili, casseroles, homemade burgers, and pasta dishes. Finely grated onion and green peppers, for example, make a wonderful addition to chilies, soups, and sloppy joes.

- **Think about prep and portions.** Grill rather than fry, and serve smaller portions. Women need 20 percent fewer calories than men to maintain their weight and half the calories of men to lose it. This means, in theory, your dinner should be half the size of your man's—unless he also needs to lose weight. As a rule, we eat too much, so begin letting your body be your hunger guide, rather than your feelings, eating history, or plate size.

- **Couch your requests positively.** Consider a typical scene at home. Your husband repeatedly brings junk food home. If you say, "Don't eat all that fattening junk food in front of me," all your husband knows is that he's not supposed to eat it in front of you. It would be better if you said, "Please eat your snacks when I'm not around," which is the behavior you really want to elicit. You'll get better results.

8. Being overweight runs in my family.

A family history of obesity increases your chances of being overweight by 30 percent. For many people, this is the result of family eating habits and exercise patterns. For example, children often learn to see cookies, candy, and other treats as rewards, or eating as a way to deal with stress or unhappiness. They view processed foods as the normal way to eat, to feed, to cope. These unhealthy eating patterns, begun in childhood, can persist into adulthood. Unlearning these patterns—substituting a hot bath or a long walk for a dish of ice cream—is part of the solution to obesity for many people.

For others, though, there may be a genetic link to obesity. Researchers have learned that some genes play a part in determining how susceptible a person is to weight gain. But genes don't doom your thighs to be forever flabby or your middle to be perpetually paunchy. You may be born with those tendencies, but this doesn't mean you are destined to be fat and sad and sick. It only means that you may have to work harder to avoid gaining weight. Three of four brothers in my family had significant and life-restricting food and weight problems—indicative perhaps of hereditary influences—but with lifestyle changes, we've been able to slim down and shape up successfully. Ask and answer the "nurture or nature" question for your food story, but don't let your answer at this moment excuse your own out-of-control eating patterns. You and any overweight relatives can start shifting those pounds by making a few small lifestyle changes in how you eat and exercise.

Don't let your excuses stand in your way of being the fittest, healthiest person you can be. As you prepare to drop the first 10 pounds, take a good, hard look at all of the excuses and justifications that will interfere with the achievement of that goal. If you value your health, stop making excuses and go after what you want.

Take 10

1. Catch yourself making excuses. How to recognize an excuse: instead of doing something, you come up with ways to explain your inaction or wriggle out of commitments that you've made to yourself.

2. Make a list of your typical excuses in your journal or *Just 10 Workbook*. Ask yourself: *Can I find a way around these? Is it worth letting these hold me back from achieving the best for myself?*

3. Find a moving meditation that you're eager to do. If physical activity feels monotonous, that's when you need to reboot and try something different.

4. Remind yourself that you're in control. Sometimes life has a way of dictating our behavior, and we forget (or at least I do) that *we* are in control. Even if I'm under too many crushing deadlines, I can still make healthful food choices.

5. Stop saying things like, "I gain weight just by looking at food." Then there's, "Once I start eating cookies, I can't stop." These are what we've come to know as "self-fulfilling prophesies." When you believe it, it is so. Changing your eating habits is not enough—you must change your thoughts, beliefs, and words.

6. Take the long view. When you run across foods you want to eat, replace excuses with words such as "I will always have another day to eat this. Looking the way I want to look and feeling great are more important right now."

7. Choices trump excuses. Once you choose to be thinner and healthier, you understand that every time you eat pizza, chips, and ice cream, you are choosing to remain overweight. If you opt to eat fruit instead of a dessert, you are choosing to become slimmer. You have used the excuse "I can't help it," but from now on you choose not to believe that.

8. Put your health first. If you don't, you're letting time slip right through your fingers. Make time for good nutrition and healthy activity. Both allow you to be more efficient at all your daily tasks. So embrace the healthy lifestyle that will take you where you want to go.

9. Don't allow fear to destroy a better life. Sometimes we worry that "this time" will end up being like all the other times we tried to lose weight and failed. This line of thought stems from fear, and it is more destructive than you can imagine. Why? Because the more you fear or worry about something, the more likely you are to act in ways that perpetuate it.

10. Start each day with positive expectations. That means expectations of success with your healthy habits and everything else you want in life. Believe you are already successful and that you are becoming more successful every day.

JUST 10 MYTH BUSTER
I CAN'T FEEL ATTRACTIVE AT
MY PRESENT WEIGHT

You may be thinking that you have to lose weight before you'll feel foxy. Not true! Don't wait until you lose weight to feel attractive. Feel attractive now! Here is a good way to start: Fix your hair, wear makeup that makes you feel special, buy clothes that flatter your body now, and walk with confidence. Love yourself now: Every day, remind yourself of at least three things you love about yourself, including your appearance, and choose different things each day. Do this several times a day; and eventually, you'll feel more attractive at your present weight. The more you can do this on a regular basis, the more you're going to notice big changes in how you feel about yourself. Also, you'll notice that you feel a bit more centered, calm, and peaceful inside. Over time, you'll feel attractive at any weight, and this genuine form of self-love will translate into everything you do, including your health and fitness habits.

CHAPTER EIGHT

STEP 8 Examine Your Battleground Beliefs

I f you asked me to name one of the biggest roadblocks to being successful in weight loss, my immediate answer would be our battleground beliefs.

What you think and feel—your beliefs—are just as important as whatever diet or exercise regimen you might initiate. In fact, clinical studies show that you can diet and exercise all you want, but if your mind and emotions aren't engaged in the weight-loss process, within two years you'll probably gain back any weight you had shed previously.

Your beliefs are often potent and can be either a positive or negative force in your life. They determine what type of work you do, what sort of home you live in, and how healthy you are. And beliefs can be used as excuses that stand in the way of success. Step 8 will help you explore what I call the four battleground beliefs and understand how they shape you:

1. Food beliefs

2. Capability beliefs

3. Life-situation beliefs

4. Relationship beliefs

Allow me to elaborate. On the road to loving yourself and weighing what you want, you will likely encounter two sides of yourself. One side that is sensible, rational, and loving—that's your loved self. From it emanates empowering beliefs, such as "I am good" and "Loving me is vital to my personal and professional success."

The other side is negative, self-critical, irrational, and unloving. It hammers your psyche with disempowering thoughts about how unlovable or unworthy you are. This kind of thinking, of course, is self-abusive. Unfortunately, we have silent, negative conversations with ourselves all the time, leading to devastating feelings of vulnerability and low self-esteem. Each of these fundamental zones of self-belief becomes a battleground on which the loved self and the unloved self go to war over food and weight. Naturally you want your loved self to win!

Some people might think the way to handle such ongoing inner conflict is just to give in to the negativity. I did that for almost 15 years. I ate what I wanted, then reduced by white-knuckle starvation or by purging. I was frequently without joy and constantly feeling defeated. That kind of life, with the two parts of me waging war for control, was deeply emotionally crippling.

You have a choice between love and hatred. They occupy the same space—one will prevail and push the other out. How good will you allow yourself to get? This is important! This is key! I want you to choose love. It's not just a matter of happy or sad, thin or fat. It's a matter of life or death. Change can begin when you enter into a new loving relationship with that person you've always been closest to: yourself.

If your beliefs do not support self-love, they must be challenged and changed. When you commit—really commit—to this change, you will mend the unloved self. This is a process, I know. But it is one you can begin while holding this book in your hands, right now. With some effort and openness, you will become someone you love and therefore someone who cares deeply about your body and succeeds with lasting weight control, health, and peace of mind. To make that happen, let's take a closer look at the four battleground beliefs.

Food Beliefs

I'm fascinated by how many people are seduced into believing a certain type of food is the reason behind their extra pounds. The French, Italians, and other cultures eat and enjoy delicious food without hysteria or much obesity, so why can't we?

We demonize and deify certain foods and have done so for quite some time. There are "good foods," "bad foods," and "really, super bad foods." And if we eat one of these, we are "terrible" or "weak" people. Eating becomes a test of moral character.

Our struggles with what we think of as good foods and evil foods have backfired. The so-called illegal foods become more and more alluring and suddenly you find yourself thinking about how you are going to sneak a bowl of pasta, which you have been told is almost as bad as doing drugs.

We're being irrational in our food beliefs. What we eat, or don't eat, certainly doesn't determine our character. As long as we view food as good or bad, we will stay hopelessly chained to unhealthy feelings toward food—and toward ourselves, really.

We're also too obsessive in our food beliefs. While nutritional labeling is a wonderful public service, I think I read those labels more intently than Moses read the Ten Commandments. There was a time when I would spend 20 minutes in the grocery store comparing the fat content of various salad dressings.

High-octane diet gurus preach on and on about food being "fuel," but who do they think they're kidding? For human beings food is much more than fuel, and to ignore that fact is just plain crazy. Food is a source of physical nourishment, yes, but it's also a source of emotional sustenance, and it's supposed to be a pleasurable experience. But when the enjoyment of sitting down to a deliciously prepared meal is overridden by fear, guilt, or anxiety, there's a problem. A healthful diet is a critically important key component, but not the be-all and end-all of a healthy lifestyle. Mentally badgering ourselves over what we have eaten, should eat, or didn't eat is not doing our minds or bodies any good.

Food is a life-giving gift and if we can be strong and make the right choices, we win more than health. We win life. Look at food in this light—approach it nonjudgmentally—and you will be freed to savor each meal rather than overeating or undereating and thus experiencing the downward spiral that goes along with those behaviors. Your body and your life will improve dramatically when you realize that you must change how you think about food, rather than the foods themselves.

Capability Beliefs

More often than not, people with food conflicts believe that they are bad or unworthy. They feel inadequate and play down their gifts, talents, and abilities. They suffer from pessimism and low self-esteem and find it challenging to love themselves with consistency and vigor. Some of the dark, disempowering beliefs here include: "I'll never be able to lose weight," "I'm a weak person," "I'll never succeed in life," "I'm a bad person because I eat too much," "I am just big boned," and "That pregnancy weight just won't come off."

Capability beliefs produce destructive "I can't" excuses. When you use the phrase "I can't" as an excuse, you send a negative, self-limiting message to your brain. Consciously, you might just pass it off as a simple excuse, but to your subconscious mind it sends a message about your abilities or inabilities. Telling yourself repeatedly that you can't do this and can't do that will have you believing that you can't do much of anything after a while.

How you view yourself and your capabilities definitely affects your weight and health. Research in the March 2005 *Journal of the American Dietetic Association* supports this assertion. Participants in a university weight-loss program all went on the same diet and exercise routine and received the same amount of support. The individuals in the group that were able to lose the most weight had a much stronger belief about being successful than their more pessimistic counterparts.

We filter so much through our capability beliefs, from the way we see ourselves in the mirror to an offhand comment we hear. If one of your capability beliefs is "I'm incompetent," you see all the experiences that support this belief and discount those that contradict it.

Everyone develops beliefs about who they are and what they can do. This is known as your self-concept. How much you like or don't like your self-concept is called self-esteem. People with low self-esteem may focus on appearance, weight, and dieting to try to feel better about themselves, but focusing on these things won't fix the bad feelings. It is important to remember that who you are and what you can accomplish in life is not defined by the shape and size of your body. It is defined by your thoughts, feelings, and actions.

Life-Situation Beliefs

Situations don't cause you to eat destructively. Rather, it's what you internalize about those various situations. If you didn't get a promotion, would you assume that your boss doesn't like you? That you're about to be fired? If you tend to interpret events in the most ego-deflating or anxiety-producing way, then your tension is at least partly self-generated.

It's common for people with food problems to use day-to-day stresses as an excuse to overeat, as I pointed out in the previous steps. "I didn't get the job I wanted, so I deserve a reward [food]." It's important to look at patterns in how you typically respond to events, and then modify or change your response to a healthier and happier one. When you do that, you develop a new understanding of how you can view yourself, treat yourself, and therefore feed yourself.

Relationship Beliefs

The satisfaction you get from relationships with family and others in your life also profoundly influences your self-concept. Too many of us lug around faulty beliefs about how we should relate to others such as the following:

- I have to be liked by everyone.
- I need to avoid conflict or anger at all costs.

- I avoid abandonment at too high a cost.

- If I show you who I really am, you won't like me.

When we hold beliefs like these, we torment ourselves. By cluttering our minds with repeated thoughts of unworthiness, we disconnect from others. All of these lead to destructive eating.

Beliefs Are a Choice

The most important thing to realize about a belief is that it's a choice. A belief is something that a person holds to be true without necessarily being able to adequately prove it.

Your battleground beliefs create your weight-loss reality, meaning that whatever you believe will affect your actions, which in turn means that your beliefs will be gradually reinforced and will persist. For example, if you believe that losing weight is hard work, you will create that as your reality. If you believe that losing weight is possible for you and that you can do it, guess what? You'll lose weight and have an easier time doing it.

So, let's cut to the chase. Here's the process I use to help people break free from battleground beliefs that do not serve them.

Identify Your Battleground Beliefs

You can notice your own negative beliefs when you catch yourself saying things such as:

- "This food is off limits because . . ."

- "I can't eat this because . . . "

- "Food helps me . . . "

- "I feel _____ when I eat _____."

- "If I go off my diet, I am _____."

- "I cannot do this because..."

- "Losing weight is..."

- "I overeat because..."

- "When things go wrong, I..."

- "I have to be liked..."

- "My relationships go bad because..."

- "I don't last long in a relationship because..."

- "Men are..."

- "Women are..."

If you find yourself repeating a negative phrase or generalization like one of the above frequently, then it's a belief. If the belief is positive, for example, you keep repeating how fortunate or successful you are, then it serves you and demonstrates self-love. However, if you find yourself repeating disempowering or unloving statements such as "I can never lose weight," you should change that belief because it's limiting you.

To change our negative beliefs, we have to know what they are. It seems like a simple step, but in reality some of our strongest beliefs lie so deep in the subconscious mind that it's challenging to bring them into consciousness. Here are some techniques that may help you do that.

Your I-Witness Account

One effective method is to create an "I-Witness Account." Here's how to do it: Take a pen and a piece of paper. Make sure nothing is going to distract you. Start writing your history with food and dieting. Brainstorm all your beliefs about food, capabilities, life situations, and relationships. Do you think some foods are "bad" and some are "good," for example? What kind of "I can'ts" are operating in your life? Which life situations—job stress, family stress, or other life stresses—cause you to overeat or not exercise? What are your beliefs about relationships? State all the beliefs you have that stop you from performing at your best ("I can't lose weight," for instance). I've included enough space in your *Just 10 Workbook* to flesh out your I-Witness Account. Getting to know your own story as fact rather than a blur of emotions is our goal.

Now explore what you've written. How did you form your beliefs? Do they provide the whole picture, or is the picture being distorted by a minor incident from your past? Is this belief based on fact or myth? If fact, what is the specific evidence that proves it? Does this belief encourage self-love? What new outlook would serve you better now?

An I-Witness Account is a confession of sorts, and as the old saying goes, confession is good for the soul. You'll uncover the past patterns that have brought you to this point so that you can forge a healthier path going forward.

Here is an excerpt of one of my client Sharon's I-Witness Accounts in which she discovered her own battleground beliefs:

> When I was a junior in high school, I went on my first diet and lost 22 pounds. On that particular diet, there were "legal" foods and "illegal" foods, so I started categorizing foods like that.
>
> My parents were happy that I lost weight. I received a lot of praise for the accomplishment and how beautiful I looked. That summer I worked in a restaurant. It was very difficult for me to control my weight in that environment. "Illegal" foods were everywhere. When I ate one, I felt enormously guilty. Then I slowly started regaining the weight I had lost. I feared my parents wouldn't love me as much if I gained weight. So early on, I developed some counterproductive battleground beliefs, and they stuck with me for a long time:
>
> - Food is either legal or illegal.
>
> - People love me only if I'm thin.

Both beliefs governed my relationship with myself and with food. The guilt that I felt over eating illegal foods and gaining weight caused me to develop an eating disorder (bulimia) that lasted from college into my early 30s. I had to get these beliefs out of my head . . . and start thinking more rationally!

Can you see how powerful and destructive such beliefs can be? Sharon went on to follow *Just 10* and lost 67 pounds. Being aware of your beliefs is the first step toward changing them—and you can change them for good just like so many others who have done what I'm asking you to do.

Examine Your Negative Battleground Beliefs

Once you have completed your I-Witness Account, read it aloud. If, while reading some statement, you get a negative feeling in your solar plexus (the area above the stomach), it means that you have just uncovered a limiting belief that is affecting your life experience.

Look over your I-Witness Account. Really study it. See where the faulty beliefs pop up. You can choose whether to keep such a belief or to eliminate it. It is up to you. Simply say to yourself that you no longer choose this belief and that from now on you will look for evidence that the opposite is true.

Keep in mind that you believe something to be true because of the "facts" that seem to support such belief. For example, if you believe that you can't lose weight, you look for the "facts" that prove you to be unsuccessful in weight loss. But by doing so, you miss out on the facts that show that this is not the case. So if you believe that you can't do it, you will only see those facts.

You have an absolute freedom to choose the way you want to live and you can choose your own beliefs and ways to behave. You should hold only yourself responsible for the person you have become. If you give this responsibility to others, you lose the power to change your life. And that's not a wise choice to make.

Family Mapping

Many of our battleground beliefs were transferred to us by our parents. If you find this to be the case, do not blame them for that. Your parents probably didn't know that their beliefs were faulty and would affect your life experience. They did what they thought was best and they shouldn't be held responsible for who you are today.

One of the best tools for breaking negative patterns is the family map, also called a genogram (pronounced: *jen-uh-gram*). I use this psychological family tree often with my patients. A proper family map reveals significant family behavior patterns—divorces, addictions, suicides, violence, and other problems—that may have affected a person's life. Many unhealthy behaviors tend to repeat themselves in families from generation to generation.

Permit me to use my own family as an example. Addiction, be it to drugs, food, gambling, or alcohol, affects two of my brothers and me. My grandparents and great-grandparents were alcoholics. I sat down and drew my family map, tracing my ancestors back a few generations. I was amazed when I looked at my map. Although addiction skipped a generation with my parents, I could clearly see that there was a perpetuating pattern of addiction in my family.

When properly drawn, the family map presents your family's psychological history as a single image and helps you identify patterns of temperament, illness, and addiction. This puts your own problems with food into context when you see that your grandmother and uncle, for example, dealt with the same problem.

We tend to believe that we choose a lifestyle of food issues or addiction, or that we're weak. But just as you may have inherited your father's blue eyes or your mother's red hair, so too can you inherit unhealthy behavior. This helps you see why there should be no guilt on anyone's part for these disorders. They were no one's fault. They didn't start with your loved one. They were passed down like silverware and china. Everyone is connected, all influencing one another all the time.

Anton Chekhov once said, "Man will become better when you show what he is like." How true. The process of reflection is healing.

When you make a conscious, more meaningful connection to your life path, it helps break the patterns and motivates change. The family map is a powerful tool for such change.

Creating Your Own Family Map

So now it's time to draw your own family map. Just follow the instructions below; and if you need more direction, go to *JUST10Challenge. com* where you can watch an instructional video to help you in this task. I've also included space and a complete legend in your *Just 10 Workbook* if you'd like to work there.

The first four steps in your family mapping cover planning and research.

1. Decide how many generations you wish to depict on your family map. You will probably want to limit it to three to four generations.

2. Gather as much information as possible to draw your family map. Talk to your relatives about your ancestors. Take notes or record the conversations so that you don't forget any details. Ask a lot of questions.

3. Get paper, a black or blue pen, a ruler, and colored markers or pencils.

4. Decide which issues you want to identify. My own map may help you decide what to look for. Each issue should have its own color. For example, use yellow to denote alcoholism, red to denote anger issues, and so forth. Or you can simply assign a letter code to each issue, as I did when I drew my family map, which is shown below.

   My codes included things like alcoholism (A), anorexia or bulimia (AB), adult child of an alcoholic (ACOA), anxiety (AX), compulsive overeating (CO), codependency (CODA), drug addiction (D), depression (DE), food addiction (F), gambling addiction (G), prescription drug addiction (RxD), smoking (S), and unresolved grief or loss (UG).

Brad Lamm Family Map

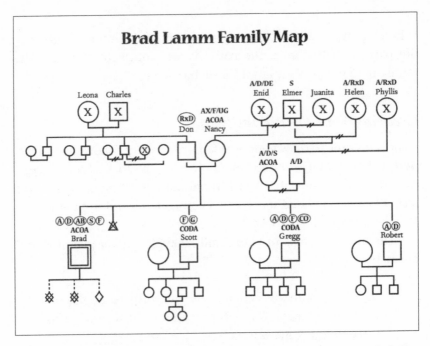

The second phase of family mapping is sitting down and drawing the map. When you draw this map, feel free to use the legends in Appendix B or make up your own based on what is appropriate for your family. For example, if you aren't Catholic, you may not need the "annulled" category that is shown in the back of the book, so you could use this line to indicate something else. Just make sure you keep a copy of what your markings mean with your family map so you can properly review it. The following steps explain the shapes and lines outlined in Appendix B:

1. Draw a double-lined square (for man) or circle (for woman) on the bottom half of the page. This shape represents you, so label it with your name. Because you are working on your own issues with this family map, you are the identified loved one (ILO).

2. Add any siblings to your right on the same part of the page, with a line connecting all of you.

3. Above you and your siblings, draw a circle and a square to represent your mother and father. Label the shapes with their names. If you know only one parent, include him or her.

4. Parallel to your parents, draw shapes to represent their siblings (your aunts and uncles). Connect all your mother's siblings with a line and all your father's siblings with another line.

5. Above your father, draw a square and circle to represent his parents (your grandparents). Do the same above your mother.

6. This step begins the coding process. If there are any divorces, indicate so with two slashes on the line connecting the couple. If there are any other types of relationships that you would like to map, use the specified lines in Appendix B.

7. Put an X through any circle or square that represents a deceased family member.

8. Finally, add the colors or letter codes that signify addictions or other issues.

You can continue to draw each generation in this manner, connecting lines and shapes for siblings, children, and other relatives. Keep all members of the same generation on the same row.

When you have finished, you should have a great overview of any recurring issues throughout the generations of your family.

Create New Empowering Beliefs

Now it's time to create some new beliefs. This is simple and fun to do. Take each of the negative beliefs you listed and turn them upside down. Take a belief like "I ate ice cream, so I am a weak person" and turn it into "I can eat ice cream in moderation and enjoy it because I have strong self-control." Basically you're stating the opposite of your negative belief.

An easy way to get started is to divide a piece of paper in two parts, write your negative beliefs on the left-hand side, and then rephrase them on the right-hand side.

Look over what you've written. Read your new beliefs aloud. Ask yourself, *What is it like having this new belief?* How does it make you feel when you read it?

Beliefs have power!

Once you're done creating your new beliefs, there's more to do.

SAYING IT FORWARD
BELIEF-CHANGING AFFIRMATIONS

Food:

- I am healthy when I stop eating when satisfied.

- I am nourished by food. It is fuel that sustains me.

- I feel energetic when I give myself the gift of healthy food.

- I feel love for myself and my family by eating purposefully.

Capabilities:

- I am great at my job.

- I am unique and special.

- I can claim gratitude in every area of my life.

- I accept myself in this present moment, without self-criticism or self-judgment, knowing that I am continuing to work on myself and do better.

Replacing Old Beliefs

We need to imprint the new beliefs into our subconscious minds. It sounds almost impossible, but it's not actually difficult at all. It takes only a little time each day, and you can actually work this into your daily practice.

In fact, your daily practice is a perfect time to reprogram your mind and imprint new beliefs. You can do it with meditations, affirmations, yoga, and so on. Affirmations are particularly powerful for changing beliefs. An affirmation is a positive statement that says exactly what it is you can do. For example: "I can control my intake of food."

Life Situations:

- I feel relaxed, focused, energetic, and enthusiastic.

- I recharge and renew myself by taking time off for play and relaxation.

- I am doing the very best I can today.

- I can choose to restart my day at any time.

- I choose to be happy.

Relationships:

- I am lovable as I am today.

- I contribute to the healthy growth of my relationships.

- I am a partner in fulfilling and nurturing relationships.

- I have friends who care about me.

Start affirming and believing the opposite of your negative battleground belief. The table on the previous pages lists some simple
affirmations, words that, when written down, spoken out loud, and
claimed, affirm the life and love and goodness inside you.

Also, describe how you are behaving when you have this new
belief ("I see myself at a restaurant, choosing healthy food, eating
small portions, and savoring each bite slowly with self-care and
affection for the beautiful person I am"). As someone with this newfound belief, take a walk and act as if you are living this new belief.
Become your new belief.

You should have faith that the opposite belief is true and that
it will color your life experience in a much richer way than the
previous belief. For example, if you used to think, *It's impossible for
me to lose weight,* you should now affirm, *I find it easy to lose weight.*
Whenever you drop a few pounds, affirm that this is the evidence of
your new belief.

Honor Your Child-Self

Another exercise people find effective for establishing new beliefs
is to honor their "child-self." Picture yourself as a small child at the
youngest age you can remember. Visualize your child-self as clearly
as possible. Or place copies of a childhood photo in which you're
younger than nine years old all around your house. (Think in the
desk drawer, or on the refrigerator door and bathroom mirror.)

When you see the image, remind yourself that the little child is
still you. Would you say the same abusive things to your child-self
as you do to your adult-self? No way! Vow to be nicer. Begin being
nicer. Cease telling her she doesn't deserve to be happy until she
loses 20 pounds. You'd never treat your own kids that way, so you
need to be more nurturing toward your most vulnerable self.

One thing I love to do is to grab my colored pencils and draw a
picture of what I want to do or be when I grow up. Remember doing
that? Try it now. Who might you be if you were unencumbered by
your battleground beliefs? What freedom might you find?

Picture that child-self in you right now. Visualize with all the
wonder and awe of that little person. Then send feelings of love

and compassion to that small you. If other less positive feelings or thoughts begin to enter, gently return your mind to thoughts of only love and compassion.

What stands behind our success is our belief system. Our beliefs guide our thoughts and our actions and determine our goals and even our relationships with others. With this step, you have all the powerful strategic artillery needed not only to navigate but to win in the difficult battlefields of self-love. When the loved self triumphs, you can become—and remain—exactly who you want to be.

Take 10

1. You have control over what you believe. Recognize your battleground beliefs and how they limit you. If you change your beliefs, you change your behavior. And once you change your behavior, you change your results.

2. Examine how your beliefs on weight loss may be holding you back: Are overweight people less lovable? Are your beliefs regarding weight loss really yours or simply ones accepted, ingrained, and reinforced over many years? How do you think losing weight would make you feel? Challenge your beliefs and you'll begin to see why you failed to reach your fitness goals in the past.

3. If you find a belief that is not serving you, simply examine it with questions like: "How true do I believe that to be?" or "Can I prove it?" and "Where did I get that idea?" These questions work remarkably well in breaking down a battleground belief.

4. Get into the habit of using affirmations to change your beliefs.

5. Changing your beliefs helps you think more positively.

Research has shown that when you think positively, your body releases endorphins that strengthen your immune system, thus improving your health and well-being.

6. Avoid using the phrase "I can't." Consider these replacements: "No, thank you," "I choose not to," "I'm not interested," "I could, but I don't want to," or "Maybe some other time." Or simply change the "I can't" to "I can," or take it one step further to "I will." These phrases will help you avoid creating negative internal feedback and creating negative beliefs about your capabilities.

7. Observe how improving your beliefs improves your life.

8. In relationships, let go of wanting approval from every Tom, Dick, and Harry or you will never have peace of mind. Help yourself reach the conclusion that people are going to be the way they are—which is often not the way you would like them to be.

9. Beliefs can produce anxiety, particularly beliefs such as "I can't cope" and "What if...?" Suppose you decided you wanted to lose weight, and then started thinking, "What if I don't stick with it?" "What if I fail again?" "What if I gain all my weight back after working so hard to take it off?" You've got a serious case of the "what ifs"! And it won't take you long to feel quite anxious. That anxiety will probably get in the way of your success. Stop trying to manage the future before it has arrived. It never works. Make a realistic plan for coping. Once you've been able to convince yourself that you can survive, even if faced with the worst possible alternative, it is easier to handle whatever happens.

10. Believe that you are not meant to be overweight, either. Your real self was made to be a healthy weight, but somehow you got off track. However, things can be corrected, and habits can change. You can get healthy. You can succeed, as long you believe it is possible.

JUST 10 MYTH BUSTER
I HAVE TO BE READY TO LOSE WEIGHT

Nearly everyone I work with makes this statement, but it's a myth with a capital M! I believe it has its origins, at least in part, in a construct called the "stages of change model," or SCM for short. SCM states that most people pass through a series of predictable phases when it comes to making a change. This theory was developed by psychologists at the University of Rhode Island and based on their study of how smokers were able to give up their habits. The model has been broadly applied to weight loss, injury prevention, and overcoming alcohol and drug problems at many treatment centers throughout the United States.

The idea behind SCM is that behavioral change does not happen in a single step. Rather, people tend to progress through different stages on their way to successful change. The myth built up around SCM is that people move through these phases most often in a self-directed way, which results in statements like, "She must be ready to change."

Working with thousands of people, what I've found is that external influences are very important in hard-to-begin behavioral change. This is often discounted by SCM. This book is an external force for change—it is challenging and inspiring. A *Just 10* buddy is an external force, as is a trainer or coach, or a support group or therapist. Bust this myth that you must plod along through stages on your own. Jump out of your current state of being, into a state of doing!

CHAPTER NINE

STEP 9 | Connect with Higher-Source Thinking

F or nearly 30 years, I abused my body horribly; it's a wonder I am even alive today. During an introspective moment, I came to a rather startling conclusion. Everything that I am, everything that I do, is the result of the body that God gave me. I've only got one, in fact—not a spare to be found—and I need to take care of it, even with the tiniest of decisions: wheat instead of white, fruit instead of candy, frozen instead of canned, water instead of juice or soda, whole instead of processed, lean instead of fatty, walk instead of sit, small instead of large, sleep instead of the late show. The list goes on and on—little decisions made moment by moment. I began to see the beauty of living a life under the influence of a loving God.

Many people find powerful and positive motivation in their faith. I happen to be one of them. I believe that there is a spiritual intelligence in every single one of us. Some call it God. Some call it Jesus. Some call it Allah or Buddha. Others call it Higher Source, Higher Power, Higher Self, or Universe.

Whatever form it takes, spirituality provides a way to make sense of our lives. The spirit in each of us is different, and we all need to find our own way of keeping in touch with it. When we find this, we can make it something that provides comfort, support, and fulfillment.

We are hardwired for spiritual connection, spiritual conversation, and spiritual intimacy. Cut off from these, we feel alone. We experience the absence of a higher power who loves us. There's no constant, guiding presence; and we are thus at great risk of engaging in, or slipping back into, the behavior that is harming us.

I know in my own life that spirituality is a force that energizes me and gives meaning to my daily life. Each day presents new opportunities and challenges, but I'm never alone. I have a community and my faith to bolster me, and a God who loves me. Spirituality enriches my life and gives me hope and inspiration, even in the darkest moments—which is why I believe that surrendering to, and connecting with, a power greater than myself is vital to my life. We need to feed our souls because we are essentially spiritual beings.

Step 9 is about making that deep, spiritual connection.

Caring for the Spirit

Your spirit refers to your deepest genuine self. It's a silent feeling that seems to say, "There is more to me than my body, thoughts, and emotions." Caring for the spirit is as important as caring for your mind and body. It is not complicated; in fact, it's pretty simple.

The easiest way to care for your spirit is to be still and spend time alone. This can be done in the form of prayer, meditation, or a moving meditation. Walking, as mentioned previously, is a wonderful tool that can get you in touch with your higher source. The rhythm of walking helps integrate the body and mind and may facilitate your ability to be more open.

Stillness is particularly important for organizing our thoughts, perceptions, and beliefs. In stillness we may find an inner place of quiet, a sanctuary that cannot be invaded by the external world. Creative inspiration often comes after prolonged stillness. Ideas and solutions to problems often make themselves known in the stillness of early morning, after several hours of sleep. Use your daily practice to be still and your journal or *Just 10 Workbook* to track progress. Explore changes and move your thoughts from mind to page.

Through solitude you can learn to create a place of quiet within that you can access whenever you need it. You can let go of the pressures of the moment and retreat to your inner place where you think through what you need to do. As you spend time alone, you come to know yourself better. You begin to differentiate between what you want and need and what someone else wants or expects you to do. You gain greater control over your own life through clarifying what you value.

When we make contact through stillness with that presence or awareness that is beyond our everyday thoughts and emotions, the result is that we think clearly and feel happier and more peaceful. And, naturally, when we have harmony on the inside, we tend to create harmonious relationships—even with ourselves!

Honor Your Temple

I do believe that we must honor our temple, which of course is our body. My faith teaches me that there is a higher source who created the world and set in motion the laws that govern it. For instance, whether or not you believe in the law of gravity, if you jumped out of an airplane without a parachute, there would be consequences. Likewise, if you violate spiritual laws of health (unhealthy food, lack of exercise, destructive habits, and so on) in caring for your body, there will be consequences. Your body chemistry will change, and disease may develop. By contrast, when we honor the body as a spiritual creation and make choices aligned with this view, we can attain a whole new level of physical and mental well-being.

Many times, when we deepen our spiritual lives, we gravitate naturally toward a more healthy diet and weight. Guided by higher-source thinking, we make wiser choices. Nutritious food, energizing exercise, and positive thoughts become staples of our everyday lives. Losing 1 pound, 5 pounds, 10 pounds, or more happens because there is an absence of struggle.

Science even corroborates that religious and spiritual people are healthier. According to research by the National Institute for

Healthcare Research (NIHR), the religious among us enjoy better health than our nonreligious friends, physically and mentally. Other studies have found that spiritual people spend less time in the hospital, are healthier, recover faster, have fewer heart attacks, and generally handle life's ups and downs in more positive ways. Spiritual people tend to live 30 percent longer and experience better physical and mental health. They also tend to have better marriages, use addictive substances less, and have stronger support systems.

As a person of faith, I definitely believe God has the ability to heal. Yes, there's the healing that occurs in the blink of the eye; but, much more often, there's healing that occurs over time. And it's here that our spirituality gives us the power to make changes. This incredible power actually alters the body's chemistry—just like a medicine might—but at a much lower cost and with no dangerous side effects.

Why does spirituality make you healthier? Experts cite a number of reasons. You benefit from active social support groups within your place of worship. Prayer and meditation may help people deal with unpleasant situations and avoid or relieve stress and depression. Religious commitment can cause positive emotions that favorably influence the immune system. Faith promotes a positive outlook that enables us to better cope with the stresses of life. Spiritual practice promotes feelings of self-control. I know that when I'm tempted to overeat or make an unhealthy choice, I hop onto my treadmill, open my favorite book, send a quick prayer heavenward, and ask my higher power for calm, so that I might refocus my thinking. Junk food doesn't stand a chance when I pray!

To take care of your temple is a loving, spiritual act with broad implications. A good example is Arthur, a friend of my family's. One day Arthur shared with me why he decided to follow his doctor's advice faithfully. "If I ever suffered a heart attack, it's not just my life that would be in disrepair; it would also put a pretty good-sized dent in the life of my wife. She'd be the one who would call 911. If I survived, she might have to push me around in a wheelchair, bathe me, and perform all of those simple, mindless tasks I do for myself now. Her life would change forever."

Arthur came to the conclusion that his health doesn't just belong to him; it belongs to his entire family. Some people say, "Hey, it's my life. I can live it any way I want." Not really. If you love those who love you, you can't live any old way you want. Whatever happens to you happens to your entire family. This is another powerful reason to honor your temple.

Many times we violate our bodies by pursuing health-destructive behaviors. In essence, we're defiling the body given to us by God. So, honor the relationships (with God and those who love you) by taking care of your body with positive health behaviors. You will be more efficient, effective, and energized. Every day, when you awaken, you'll feel the joy that comes with realizing that life is an incredible gift for those who choose to live it wisely.

Make Mealtimes Special

We know that food guarantees our physical survival. It also sustains us emotionally and spiritually by providing regular opportunities for relaxation, celebration, and connection. You see this in all faiths.

One of the most profound ways to connect to higher-source thinking is to make mealtimes special with a blessing and calm, reflective eating. I have always been open to prayer, even if it has sometimes seemed like a mysterious, otherworldly activity. But even in my darkest periods I always managed to give thanks for my food before a meal.

Here's a snapshot of how this helps me. One recent evening with friends, I came to the dinner table at the end of my rope. It had been a long day, and there were still many tasks ahead. The last-minute premeal tension crackled through the air as I darted around, opening the refrigerator, reaching for the lettuce, slamming a cupboard shut, juggling a handful of silverware along with my iPhone.

In the midst of all this, I dropped a glass pitcher of iced tea. Glass and liquid flew everywhere. I sat down at the table with a black cloud over my head. I wish one of my friends had turned the mood

around with the kind of funny comment that puts these stressful moments in perspective, but that didn't happen. Nevertheless,
something wonderful shifted the mood anyway. I bowed my head
and said, "Thank you for the food and the people at this table."
But I not only said it, I also meant it. For one moment the chaos
stopped; the noise was pushed aside. I felt my heart stop racing, my
face cool down, and my ears get less red. It was a calming moment,
what I call saving grace.

I see a desperate need in today's culture to reestablish calmness
around food. We are missing the celebration with which we come
together as a community to eat, the celebration and enjoyment of
working together and nourishing our bodies with thankfulness for
the food we receive.

I believe that the idea of "mindful eating" is a tool to bring
ourselves back to balance. Mindfulness means being fully aware
within the present moment. When you practice mindful eating,
you pay attention to your body's subtle and natural cues, specifi-
cally the ones that say "feed me" and "that's enough." It's appealing
because it's a mind-set instead of a meal plan. And it can help you
lose weight.

I'll elaborate: A lot has been written about some of the more
tedious practices of mindful eating: meticulously observing the prop-
erties of your food, slowly lifting the fork to your mouth, chewing
each bite thoroughly, visualizing its journey to your stomach, and
all that. But even if you don't have the time (or, frankly, the inclination) to go through this process every time you sit down to a meal,
it's still possible to lose weight using some of the methods that make
the approach successful. Deana, a client I coach, experienced this firsthand, after losing four pounds in two weeks simply by noticing when
she was hungry and never eating past the point of being satisfied. She
also set up "speed bumps" during her meals: putting down her utensils
between bites and alternating her focus between food and conversation. These gave her body the necessary 20 to 30 minutes to register
the I'm-feeling-full message. If you eat when you're hungry and stop
when you're full (really satisfied, not the feeling of full, mind you),
you'll have an easier time keeping your weight in check.

The point is to make mealtimes special and peaceful. Don't wolf your food down. Pace yourself. Sit down to a table carefully set with china and silverware. Light a candle. Decorate your table with flowers. Offer a prayer of thanks for the meal. Eat carefully, consciously, and mindfully.

Healing Forgiveness

Another spiritual tool that connects you to higher-source thinking is forgiveness. Life brings us all kinds of personal hurts. When you feel wronged by someone, it can be hard to get past the hurt, and not everyone is willing to try. But people who hang on to anger, grudges, disappointments, and thoughts of revenge pay a high price with their physical health and emotional energy. They are at much greater risk of developing chronic ailments, such as heart disease. Unforgiveness and its psychological baggage of hostility and bitterness can put people at risk for mental illness, too, such as depression and anxiety, not to mention stress disorders and related physical ailments.

Bolstered by evidence that vengefulness could carry heavy physical health risks, more scientists are taking a serious look at forgiveness and how it affects the whole person. A small but growing body of evidence also suggests that forgiveness—particularly for severe hurts—plays a role in lowering depression and anxiety. It's also been linked to small increases in self-esteem and self-love.

Even the human body practices forgiveness. There is proof all around us. This is why a woman in her 40s who has barely worked out in the last 20 years can decide to start training and run a marathon. This is why a pack-a-day smoker can give up cigarettes and start breathing better in only a matter of weeks. This is why someone who has been eating fatty foods his whole life can eat healthier for a month and see his cholesterol spiral down by his next doctor visit.

Forgiveness has long laid the foundation for spiritual well-being. Most faiths believe that we were not designed to hold on to anger, revenge, bitterness, and resentment. When we do, it's destructive to our being, leading to a slow and insidious breakdown of the entire system. For when we hate others, we feel the pain of hating over and over again. It leaves you emotionally exhausted. Dwelling on the situation gives it—and the person who wounded you—too much power. The only way to true healing is to forgive and let go.

Forgiveness is something you do purely for yourself. You are not doing it for the person who has transgressed or wronged you, and you don't even need to express forgiveness to the person in question. This doesn't mean you have to like what he or she did, but you must emotionally release it. When you're ready to do that, mentally rewrite the story of what happened. Instead of seeing yourself as a victim, cast yourself as a strong person who's triumphed over a painful experience. Picturing yourself in a place of victory gives you increased confidence to deal with future disappointments. So don't let the experience drag you down. The consequences of not forgiving and staying stuck are too high.

My client Gene saw firsthand how holding on to a grudge turned a stressful job situation into a full-blown weight problem. He gained 30 pounds in a three-month period and admitted to his doctor that it was due to stress eating. Gene was a reporter for a daily newspaper in a major city, and his job was stress laden even on a good day. Still, he had no serious problems until he felt his boss, a senior editor, began to treat him unfairly by making capricious changes, demanding he redo approved work, and requiring that he still make deadlines. Gene began eating mounds of junk food to cope.

At first, Gene thought it was just the stress that made him binge; but when he talked it over with me, we realized that it was the anger. "I knew I had to forgive those who mistreated me, or I would suffer even more," he admitted.

Actively holding on to destructive emotions or thoughts that surround an injury takes you down a dangerous path, potentially leading from anger to bitterness and even consuming hatred. In Gene's case, his anger took him over the edge into destructive eating.

"I had always thought anger was a part of how I coped, and I finally realized it didn't have to be," Gene said. "I could have avoided a lot of life's pain if I'd learned to forgive a long time ago. I thought that by hating that editor, I was paying him back, but I was just hurting myself."

The awareness of his unforgiveness started him on the path to healing and controlling his self-destructive patterns.

Genuine forgiveness is hard work, not the stuff of doormats and wallflowers as the American culture of rugged individualism and competition would have us believe. Despite the difficulty of genuinely forgiving, increasing evidence suggests that the work is well worth the effort. In forgiveness, you exchange anger, bitterness, hatred, depression, and perhaps health problems for joy, peace, and freedom. Not a bad trade by any standard.

When It's Time to Act

I'll tell you a secret for making your life work—sort of a "duh" secret because it's so obvious: take action. Einstein said, "Nothing happens until something moves." We can't simply pray and think about what we want. We must act with intention.

What do you want? What are you committed to? What are your priorities? What do you want to achieve? Take out a piece of paper and write down your commitments. Are you committed to your family, to your kids, to living as an example of engaged spirituality? Do your priorities reflect those commitments? If I were to walk around with you for a day or two, what would I say your priorities are? And yes, you should pray and meditate on these desires.

Once you're clear on what they are, and you've been in prayer or meditation about them, it's time to take action. Spirituality is action. If you've ever said of someone, "I like her spirit," you are not describing passivity. You're describing someone who is engaged in the vital activity of living. To pray or meditate, and then not act, can be so counterproductive—like dreaming a pleasant dream, but never waking up to life. A lot of people talk about losing weight, yet don't do anything about it. Until you do it, you won't be happy. Act on your prayers and meditation, even if only in simple ways, like enjoying a nourishing meal or taking a short walk around the block.

As we come to the end of this step, know that spirituality is different for everyone. But there is a unifying principle in all forms of spiritual practice: personal well-being and proper eating and exercise are linked. We can improve our physical world through practice living in our spiritual world.

Take 10

There are many ways you can communicate with your higher source on any need. Just decide the forum and have a serious talk. If it's your weight that's bothering you, ask that the burden be lifted. Say something like this: "I need to lose weight, and I'm having trouble. I need help. And I believe that if you help me, then I know I'll have a chance." Here are 10 ways to connect with your higher source:

1. Prayer

2. Meditation (including guided meditation at *Just10Diet.com*)

3. Reading spirit-feeding books, biblical verses, or other religious texts

4. Worship in a church, mosque, synagogue, temple, or other place of spirit

5. Moving meditations

6. Daily practice

7. Small groups in religious studies

8. Yoga

9. Faith-based weight-loss support groups

10. Pilgrimages to holy places

JUST 10 MYTH BUSTER
SPIRITUALITY ALWAYS
INVOLVES A DEITY

Your spiritual life doesn't have to be defined by a deity. Spirituality can also be an attitude: It can be that feeling of love that connects us all; serving others, particularly the less fortunate; or the state of being happy enough with what one has or is, not desiring something more or different. Or spirituality might be a sense of gratitude and hope that recognizes even the little things in life as special events. At its essence, spirituality is a sense of purpose in life—a connection between the individual and the sacred.

CHAPTER TEN

STEP 10

Pay It Forward

I f you've been living the first nine steps and following the *Just 10* 30-Day Plan, your bathroom scale should read 10 pounds lower than when you started. Congratulations! Now you'll make a new *Just 10* goal weight and do more of what you've done.

What will it take to keep going, to reach your ultimate goal, to maintain the changes, and to have a healthy relationship with food? Sure, there are tips like stay active, watch calories and portions, notice fat grams, and know your numbers—your weight, your waist, your cholesterol. The longer you cleave to your new patterns—and find success in them by eating natural, body-honoring foods—the easier it will be to stick to it. The bottom line is that a shift in spirit, so important to maintaining lasting change, has already begun. You are truly retraining yourself inside and out.

But there are no simple solutions, because it can be a daily struggle to overcome the temptation to overeat. Looking back at the thousands of people I've helped, those who sustain the weight loss are the ones who have addressed the inside job. They've had a shift in spirit that led them to a renewed sense of self and a commitment to self-care. They have come to love themselves in a healthy, new way.

But there is one more step, and I think it works miracles. Pay it forward is Step 10.

Step 10 is about helping others, no matter where you are in your journey. As poet and novelist Lily Hardy Hammond (who lived during the turn of the last century) once said, "You don't pay love back; you pay it forward."

Numerous 12-step programs show that addicts and alcoholics get well by developing the habit of helping others. In the process, they learn that no matter how valuable their support is to others, they get as much or even more out of it. They're living proof of the phrase "To keep it, you've got to give it away." This is another way of saying pay it forward.

If we want serenity, we can try to increase serenity in others. If we want more faith, we help others grow theirs. If we want hope, we can encourage hope in someone else. If we want health, we must help others achieve it.

Good acts—acts of kindness, generosity, and helpfulness—spread easily. In a study published in the March 8, 2010, online edition of the *Proceedings of the National Academy of Sciences*, researchers from the University of California at San Diego and Harvard University provided the first laboratory evidence validating that helpful, cooperative behavior is contagious and that it spreads from person to person. When people benefit from kindness, they pay it forward by helping others, and this creates a cascade of cooperation that influences dozens more in a social network.

In the study, the researchers show that when one person gives money to help others, the recipients are more likely to give their own money away. This creates a domino effect in which one person's generosity spreads first to three people and then to the nine people that those three people interact with in the future, and then to still other individuals in subsequent waves.

As I read this study, I got to thinking that if we started unselfishly paying forward what we know about losing weight, we might end the obesity epidemic in our time.

I believe with all my heart that if we can develop the habit of giving all of these things away—love, knowledge, compassion, health, time, talents, and more—we will experience them more and more inside ourselves. I know that whenever I am out of balance, I turn my attention to offering someone a hand, whether through a phone call, an e-mail or text, or an in-person visit. Nothing takes my mind off myself like turning to another who could use some love and help.

People who pay it forward can keep their weight off—and without any of that grit-your-teeth-and-do-it kind of behavior. Let me share two stories that illustrate this.

Yvonne's Story

I met Yvonne many years ago at a Quaker retreat in Costa Rica. A fit, athletic-looking brunette with dancing green eyes, Yvonne was charming, intelligent, soft spoken, and most of all...calm. We immediately struck up a friendship and started going to some of the retreat events together, and she told me about herself.

One night 10 years ago, Yvonne was strolling out of a movie, chatting with her 12-year-old son, Wes, about the evening, when suddenly she was overcome with dizziness. She got to her car, leaned against the door, and waited for it to pass. Luckily for Yvonne, her concerned son had other ideas. With worry in his heart and soul that he might lose his mom, Wes insisted that she go to the emergency room. There doctors told Yvonne that she had just experienced a mild heart attack.

Yvonne admitted she'd been having mild chest pains for six or seven months at that point, but she thought it was just job-related stress. "Heart disease was the last thing on my mind," Yvonne told me. "I didn't have high blood pressure or high cholesterol. But, yes, I had always struggled with my weight, staying 30 to 50 pounds above the norm for me."

After several tests, doctors discovered a small blockage in a tiny artery. Yvonne, who was only 47 at the time, had open-heart surgery to remove the blockage, but there was the looming question about the role her weight might be playing (especially given the absence, in her case, of other significant risk factors). Her doctors were adamant: lose the weight and keep it off.

The mandate sounded like a tall order—and it was. Like all of us, Yvonne had tried to lose weight so many times in the past—and she had succeeded, but only temporarily. She could never keep it off. She was a binge eater, often consuming boxes of cookies or pastries in a single sitting. The behavior left her feeling that she was worthless and that life was hopeless.

Her brush with death forced some major changes in her life: keeping high-calorie junk food out of the house; passing up second and third helpings of mashed potatoes, gravy, and desserts; and getting more consistent exercise.

All of it worked, but problems of weight gain come from within. To stay healthy, Yvonne knew she had to make emotional and spiritual shifts in the way she viewed herself and approached the world. Yvonne persisted on her journey of recovery and, in doing so, came back with a fierce energy that transformed her life. She lost weight, lost her destructive habit, and lived each and every day as though it, and her entire life, really did matter.

When I asked Yvonne exactly how she was able to exchange a life of insanity for one filled with many more moments of peace, serenity, and self-love, Yvonne shared her philosophy. "I try to help others," she said with a smile.

Yvonne explained to me that she constantly talks to and helps scores of other people who are struggling with food and weight issues. Yvonne goes to counseling centers, hospitals, churches, schools—wherever there are people dealing with weight problems. She candidly shares the challenges she has faced in reconciling her relationship with food with the realities of living positively.

"I began living in the solution," Yvonne told me. She learned that she could take the power out of her self-defeating behavior by speaking out and helping others. And there will always be people to help.

Scott's Story

Scott is my brother. Three years older than me, he was often my protector. When I'd get bullied, he'd put a stop to it. Among the four Lamm boys, he was always the thin one and by far the most athletic. There was never a sport or activity he wouldn't dive right into with success.

Scott ate whatever, whenever, however. The list was long. Chips, dips, candy, sodas, and fast food. A normal lunch for him would consist of an entire bag of Doritos and a two-liter bottle of Pepsi. He'd never gain an ounce because he was so active and played a lot of sports.

Fast-forward 30 years. He showed up at a family reunion in 2009. I was shocked by his weight gain. Scott had put on 35 pounds over a long period of time, but then packed on 70 more over a short spell. He confessed that he was addicted to fast food, and would easily scarf down 2,500 calories in a single sitting.

"I can't stop," he confided to me.

Standing just shy of 5 foot 9, Scott had ballooned to nearly 275 pounds, with a 44-inch waist. This was a far cry from the 170 pounds and 31-inch waist he sported in high school. I hugged him. I told him I loved him and gave him an invitation to change. I gently said that he didn't have to live like that anymore. He could change his relationship with food if he was willing to let me show him how. I challenged him to live the 10 steps and focus on the first 10 pounds. Scott was in so much physical and emotional pain that he committed to follow through. If the body truly is the temple, then it was time to clean the house. And so he began the work of self-discovery.

I assured him that he'd have to focus on only 10 pounds at a time. I promised that if he did just that, he'd make it and his life would change in amazing ways. Scott had to relearn when to eat (only in response to actual hunger), how much (only what he needed for fuel—meaning a lot less food), and when to stop (when he was satisfied). When he wasn't hungry, instead of snacking, he worked on himself through his daily practice, regular affirmations, and moving meditations.

Scott's greatest reservation was that his travel schedule didn't allow for a healthy eating plan. I promised him his schedule would allow for it—if he would—and we got to work.

Scott grabbed onto the *Just 10* plan as though it were a life preserver. It kept him afloat when he ached to go back under. Working with a *Just 10* buddy (me), Scott learned to love himself again by writing about his past, appreciating his body, understanding his cravings and triggers, and pulling his thoughts out of some very dark places.

When Scott began his program, he asked me about Alli, an over-the-counter, FDA-approved drug that helps the body rid itself of consumed fat. He wanted to find out more about its safety and side effects because he was having a hard time fighting his cravings for high-fat, nutrient-poor food. I have had clients use Alli in the past, and many found that it helped keep the fat in check. I suggested that Scott try it to temper his desires for those foods that "talked" to him from the store shelf—the chocolate, the chips, and the candy bars. While Alli isn't part of my own food story, I think it can prove useful in certain cases. Please discuss its use with your doctor to make sure that it's safe for you.

Ultimately the weight dripped off Scott, like a candle burning itself down. Along the way, his cholesterol went down, and he was able to go off cholesterol-lowering drugs.

The last 20 pounds were tough, but he worked his way through them. With persistence and dedication—not to mention his new habit of always carrying a Cinch bar with him—he managed to maintain his internal eating clock on the road and live a more healthy life in general. Over 17 months, and without any surgery, Scott lost almost 100 pounds.

Scott did the work and moved through the phases I call: Mend – Move – Maintain. He's now at a healthy weight—edging closer and closer to the 170 pounds he used to weigh—and he's enjoying the benefits of a body that reflects the love he's chosen to show it.

Scott is also paying it forward. He works earnestly and passionately as a weight coach at Change Institute to help others peel off their own fat suits and find wellness. Who better than a guy who has lost 100 pounds and found himself again? While Scott's story is uniquely his own, millions share his struggle of out-of-control eating that causes much emotional and physical pain. And now he is sharing his solutions.

He told me recently, "Helping people, especially with their weight . . . whether it's simply listening to people who feel there is no hope, or helping someone figure out how to get healthy . . . well, after all these years, I've found my calling."

I believe people are alive today because of Scott.

How can you do what Scott is doing? How do you live out a principle like pay it forward?

How to Pay It Forward

There are many ways. Think about doing something for another person. Or pick a cause you want to support and volunteer your time and talents to help make a difference. I know what you might be thinking: you'd like to volunteer, but you're too busy. Sure, we're all busy with family and professional obligations. But being busy is just a matter of reprioritizing your time. Yes, it is important to take care of us first, and paradoxically, helping others is one way to do that, as long as you make time for it. When we volunteer or help others, we're giving ourselves many physical, mental, and emotional benefits.

Again, science agrees. Research shows that you can experience the same physiological changes when you help others as you do when you exercise. Heart rate and breathing decrease and feel-good endorphins are released—all of which power up the immune system.

In a landmark study on volunteering, researchers found that those who helped regularly were physically healthier than people who volunteered only once a year. The regular helpers reported fewer illnesses from colds, allergies, and asthma; less depression; fewer aches and pains; and a sense of calmness and well-being.

In another fascinating study, investigators at the University of Michigan followed 2,700 people for more than a decade to see how volunteering affected their health and found that these selfless acts were linked to a lower death rate.

Although scientists cannot draw definite conclusions as to why volunteering is so powerful, it is widely believed that working together toward a common good seems to activate reward-related areas of the brain. Other studies report that volunteering is linked to social ties and trust. The result: the feel-good boost that motivates people to do even more good to feel even better. I've been asked again and again how to build self-esteem. The answer is easy: Do valuable things. It's good to be good to others.

Or as Ralph Waldo Emerson summed it up: "It is one of the most beautiful compensations in life that no man can truly help another without helping himself."

There are just so many ways to pay it forward. When you do, you'll find new meaning in life, a meaning that transcends your own needs. It is through caring, sharing, teaching, showing by example, and investing the very best we have to offer that we find what is most precious in life. By helping others, we help ourselves. There is no scarcity of goodness and grace. You will always keep what you have when you give it away.

Take 10

1. Help those who need extra motivation get to the gym or start a moving meditation (if they want help). Help educate others who also struggle with obesity—at your church, in workshops, in your neighborhood, or at work. Any of these activities can give you a new sense of purpose and keep you active, too. You now have the power to help in the fight against obesity.

2. Host a meeting. Or, if you're a business owner, open your place of business for people who want to start a weight-loss group.

3. Volunteer at a local charity. For instance, at your local humane society, you could walk, play with, or wash dogs. You'll love it because you're helping out and getting exercise. Or consider helping out at a local hospital, or as a responder for a suicide hotline.

4. Donate. If you're financially able, send a check to a charity or organization of your choice.

5. Organize a food drive. My brother Gregg's church in Newberg, Oregon, saw a growing need in their small town. Many folks were going to bed hungry. This past October they collected more than seven tons of food to distribute

in their community. They call this now-annual food drive: FEED THE NEED. What would you call your food drive?

6. Get into the business. Many personal trainers are formerly overweight people. It's not volunteering, but it's another way of paying it forward. Gena is a good example. Several years ago, she didn't look like she'd ever be a typical health-club employee. But at 5 foot 4 and 179 pounds, she did look like someone who could benefit from a health-club membership. Gena eventually lost 50 pounds through a plant-based diet, weight training, and therapy. Her lifestyle change motivated her to leave her job as a lawyer behind to become certified as a personal trainer. Today she's one of the most popular trainers at Equinox Health Club in New York City—because she understands what her clients are facing.

7. Pitch in against childhood obesity. It is now estimated that one in five children in the United States is overweight, putting them on the road to lifelong chronic conditions such as diabetes and heart disease. Children have not chosen a life of obesity for themselves. Changes in our society over the past few decades make it more difficult for families to make healthy choices. Too many families live in areas without affordable access to healthy foods and without safe places for children to be physically active. This is something we can and must change.

8. Be a Big Brothers Big Sisters mentor. Model healthy living for a young person. Setting an example for someone is very powerful. If a young person sees you eating a healthy diet, they are more likely to start eating a healthy diet, too. If they see you enjoying exercise, they might become more active, too. Also, volunteer at a summer fitness camp for kids, or help out with recreational programs for children at a local gym or YMCA.

9. Be a healthy role model in your family. This is a wonderful way to pay it forward. If you want your kids to do healthy

things, let them learn from you. This is called modeling. Kids don't come into this world with good health habits. They have to learn them, and the way kids learn is by example. If your eating and exercise habits are poor, your children's probably will be, too. Do things like cook healthy meals together. Slow down and gather together for meals. Let them help you by doing the dishes! Once you get them involved, they get more interested.

10. Make physical activities a family affair. Try biking, hiking, swimming, or skating as a family. Play with your kids regularly in vigorous outdoor games. There is an old saying that still rings true today: Our children are watching us live, and what we are shouts louder than anything we can say.

JUST 10 MYTH BUSTER
YOU HAVE TO BE RICH OR
RETIRED TO VOLUNTEER

The truth is, there is room for all of us in the world of volunteering. The gratification that comes from helping others is humongous. It generates that little glow inside that provides us with a feeling of what it is to give without return or reward. As a volunteer you bring distinct life experiences, different occupational skills, languages, and new perspectives to those in need. It's time to ask yourself what you have to offer!

Change Begins

felt called to write this book. I wanted to instill ideas and inspire action. The tug was deep and urgent: DO THIS NOW. And so I did. But a diet book is only as good as the person acting on it. Even equipped with a strong plan, it all comes back to you.

The effectiveness of all the science, soul, experience, and hope I've poured into *Just 10 Lbs.* depends on what you do now. Ups and downs will come, but so will living lighter—both spiritually and physically—if you take the *Just 10* steps to heart. Everyone I've worked with who has broken free from their negative patterns shares one thing in common: each has had a shift in spirit that allowed them to walk out of crisis and into the sunlight.

Remember, you needn't eat from a place of emotional binge-ing ever again because now you know that you're really hungry for more than food. You're hungry for sustainable change, and that change begins with pledging to follow the *Just 10* program.

So, with faith and love, join me now in that pledge.

Here we go . . . together.

Onward,

Brad

Just 10 — The 30-Day Plan

M ost of us start off a new fitness or health program totally gung ho, but after a couple of weeks, our dedication wanes, we get bored, or we decide we're not getting a quick enough payoff for our effort. So we quit.

To keep that from happening, I've broken down the principles in this book into a simple 30-day plan that allows you to focus on one single task or challenge per day. The plan includes advice for incorporating the steps into your life, affirmations to use in your daily practice, and a menu plan (starting on page 185) to help you build new routines around food. Each morning, read your daily advice and affirmations, and then flip to the menus. This 30-day plan will help you create new habits, so your new lighter, self-loving lifestyle can grow and take root. It really works. And I promise I haven't assigned anything you're not capable of!

Remember, you're never alone in this effort, no matter how you may feel at any given moment, minute, hour, or day. I'm in it with you. Grab on to this 30-day plan with me. It will psych you up to eat right, get active, and invite calm into your life.

Start your 30 days tomorrow, and look forward to giving yourself this treat for the month.

Prior to Starting

I'm sure you've heard the expression "Get your ducks in a row," and here's your place to do just that. These tips will help you reach your *Just 10* goal in short order.

- **Plan ahead.** Clear your kitchen, car, office, and other locations of binge food. Make the areas in which you dwell, safe spaces. Out with the craving foods, and in their place, stock your pantry and fridge with foods recommended on the food plan: eggs, chicken breasts, fish, vegetables, apples, extra-virgin olive oil, lemons, salad dressing, various and richly colored greens, and so forth. If a food is not on your list, don't eat it!

- **Schedule it.** Begin to schedule the time you need for your daily practice and physical activity, and focus on how you will accomplish each of these easy—and enriching—tasks. You'll feel better for it, and I hope you'll want to incorporate most of these ideas into your everyday routine.

- **Take your vitamins.** Introduce a multi-vitamin into your morning routine to make sure you cover your vitamin and mineral bases.

- **Use your journal or *Just 10 Workbook*.** This will help you document your progress, your plan, and your path as it unfolds. Weigh yourself, and record your numbers in your journal—remember to write down your current weight and your *Just 10 Lbs.* goal weight. Don't get overwhelmed. Focus only on the 10. In the workbook you'll find pages with exercises for you to do, space for food planning and journaling, as well as spots to track your progress. Watch the numbers change for the better as you begin to alter your mood and your food and your habits.

DAY 1

Start the *Just 10* Love-Centered Food Plan. Review Chapter 1 and then head to page 185 to see the first menu in the 30-day plan. Drink plenty of water throughout the day, too. The easiest way to make sure you drink your eight glasses of water during the day is to have a full one-liter bottle at your desk. And drink water with your meals and snacks. Also:

- Fill out the questionnaire to determine your eating style; write down strategies that resonate with you.

- Eat a wide variety of foods during the day.

- Commit to your meals for the day, and don't deviate from the plan.

- Listen to your body's signals of satiety and hunger.

- Use food to fill the emptiness in your stomach, not your heart.

- Gravitate toward foods that are unprocessed and natural.

- Eat with the awareness that you are nourishing your body with life-affirming, body-honoring foods.

DAILY AFFIRMATION: The past is gone. Today is full of possibilities to change my weight and my health. With every bite, I'm giving my body the energy it needs to work and repair.

DAY 2

Begin to think about your daily practice: What will it look like? Will I pray, meditate, visualize, or do something else? What are the intentions I will set for my day? You might start your daily practice by visualizing the 24 hours ahead: eating healthfully, moving your body, or standing in gratitude for all you have. Create a sacred place in your home for your practice. Clear out any clutter to release stagnant energy. Burn a scented candle to fragrance the air and bring a

new atmosphere into the room. Fill it with objects you find calming and inspirational. Start by spending just a few minutes there to
experience what it feels like. Twenty minutes is ideal, but even five
minutes of solitary meditation or relaxation will help restore your
spirit. Beginning with today, start each day with your daily practice.
Determine what your life will look like each day. If you see your day
going smoothly, you will create such a day.

DAILY AFFIRMATION: I relax in the stillness and take a few deep
breaths. Breathing in, I envision a perfectly healthy day of better
food, more activity, and peace of mind. Nothing can disrupt the
serenity I carry within me.

DAY 3

Turn your wholehearted attention to how you will move your body.
Decide on forms of exercise that are appropriate for you and do one
today. Make those activities moving meditations. It's fine—and
indeed I encourage it—if your routine varies. One day you might
choose to take a brisk walk. On another, you might work out with
weights. Another time you can make it a no-weight workout. Or,
you may decide to clean your house to music, or connect with
nature by gardening. Be open to the many ways you can improve
your health by varying your activities. By focusing on simply moving more, rather than planning elaborate exercise sessions, you will
improve your fitness level and be in a better mood.

DAILY AFFIRMATION: There will be many opportunities to move
today. Taking action refreshes and renews me, and I feel vitally alive.

DAY 4

We have all formed habits of thought about ourselves and our bodies. Some of these thoughts add to our well-being, others detract
from it. Sometimes we're not tuned in to our negative thoughts;
so we don't realize how they keep us from being healthy, happy,

and successful. Thoughts of body hatred, failure, or negative battleground beliefs have an undesirable effect. To say "I am weak" or "I am ugly" or "I can't" attaches these conditions to us, and the more often we repeat them, the truer they become. Today, take stock of your thoughts and beliefs. If they are habitual, decide to change the character of your thinking. You can do this with a spiritual approach, with relaxation, positive programming of your mind, or even with a counselor. Reassure yourself about something specific that troubles you. For example, say, "I am great at my job," "I have a lot of friends who care about me," "I am a good guy, who is working hard to make change," or "I'm lovable just the way I am today."

DAILY AFFIRMATION: I part with my old pattern of thinking to make way for the new. I breathe out the old and breathe in the new. I visualize each piece of negative self-talk in my mind as a balloon that I release to the sky, never to be seen again.

DAY 5

I once read that after four days of doing things "right," we get a little weary and want to slip back into our old habits. I don't know if this is true. But if you're feeling this way, make a list of 25 non-food-related activities to do to enhance your life, such as: exercising, reading, pursuing a favorite hobby, listening to music, communicating with friends via Facebook or email, making a gratitude list, or soaking in a hot bath. Keep your list handy.

DAILY AFFIRMATION: The actions I take today are key. They direct my steps, either forward or backward. I just have to move my feet in a new direction and make the right choices, and I will reach my goal.

DAY 6

Today, you'll "ID" your food triggers and figure out ways to prevent unhealthy overeating. Think about your triggers. Are they about people, places, things, pressures, or all of the above? Are they excuses you're using to justify behavior? Strategize how to gain mastery over them. Take a clean page in your journal or *Just 10 Workbook* and divide it into two columns with My Personal Food Triggers on the left and My Strategies for Mastery on the right. Then make lists under each one. It's a handy tool for mapping out an effective game plan. Do this when you feel tempted.

DAILY AFFIRMATION: I may encounter an obstacle today; maybe even more than one. I have stepped around them before, and I do so again today.

DAY 7

Being fit feels different. In your journal or *Just 10 Workbook*, list all the many feel-great changes you have noticed over the past six days, no matter how small they seem. Frame it as your *Just 10* gratitude list. Some examples: more energy and greater stamina, better sleep, greater confidence, less stress and anxiety, or a better outlook on life.

DAILY AFFIRMATION: With each day, positive choice, and new awareness, I am moving, growing, changing, and loving myself more deeply than ever.

DAY 8

It's easy to get obsessed with what we don't like when we look in the mirror, especially since we're surrounded 24/7 by images of people with perfectly toned bodies and flat abs. Your relationship to your body is the first relationship you have, and it's the most important one. To work on loving your body more, do three things today to improve your appearance. Get a new haircut, buy a new suit, or have a manicure, for example. Revisit your body map, and if you didn't do one before, return to page 66 and create one now. You'll feel better, inside and out.

DAILY AFFIRMATION: I look for beauty today, in myself and in my life, and I find it.

DAY 9

Take this day to enjoy the satisfaction of performing a single act of kindness: write a thank-you note to someone who recently helped you with even a minor task, or pick out a small, meaningful gift for someone special in your life. Step 10 tells us that we must pay it forward to keep it. Practice this step today.

DAILY AFFIRMATION: Every day is a chance to exchange gifts. I give, and I receive.

DAY 10

Try something new today. I recommend yoga. Get a DVD, tune in to a yoga class on television, or visit *JUST10Challenge.com* for my dear friend Bryant Stiney's *Yoga for Beginners* videos. Try it for at least 20 minutes. It will help stretch your muscles and relax your body. Commit to doing yoga or some form of stretching at least twice a week. This will increase your flexibility, which is a key component of fitness. Yoga allows you to combine stretching with self-care and relaxation.

DAILY AFFIRMATION: I have the courage to try something new today. It holds the promise of growth.

DAY 11

Connect with someone you love. Go out to lunch or have dinner together. If you live alone, play with your pet or call a friend. Studies have shown that bonding with others, including animals, decreases rates of depression and boosts the immune system. For support in other ways, look into a support group experience. Support enriches our lives. The experiences shared among friends help us live more fully. It's no accident that certain people have been drawn together. What you have will help them and vice versa.

DAILY AFFIRMATION: The remedy for loneliness is connectedness. Today I reach out to others with whom I can share my life. They lighten my burdens and I lighten theirs.

DAY 12

Learn to value your body by becoming aware of the hard work it does for you every day, every hour, every second. One way to do this is to concentrate on one particular part of your body while you're doing something productive. For example, focus on your feet, and ask them questions such as: "Hey feet, how many steps have you walked today? Thank you for that!" Or ask your hands: "How many things have you carried, pulled, pushed, lifted, turned, squeezed and lovingly touched during the past couple of years? How many pages of a book have you turned, how many children or sick people have you held?" Do the same for all your body parts, for your back, your knees, your eyes, your nose, your heart, your lungs, and your brain. Have a conversation with yourself. Be good to your body, and your body will be good to you.

DAILY AFFIRMATION: Regardless of any opinion or appearance to the contrary, I know that my body is designed to serve me; healing, renewing, purifying, and making me whole.

DAY 13

Go to the grocery store today and buy at least one fruit and one vegetable you've never tried, or haven't had in a long time. Look for produce that is in season. Consider adding the local farmers' market to your routine. Prepare the new food lovingly and eat with gratitude. Know that you are honoring your body with this choice.

DAILY AFFIRMATION: I make the right nutritional choices with ease and confidence, because I get energy and health from body-honoring foods.

DAY 14

Give your body some extra-special attention today. Pampering your body need not be expensive. A good massage, a bubble bath, a homemade facial, a relaxation or visualization exercise, a long walk or bike ride—all of these activities are expressions of your love for your body.

DAILY AFFIRMATION: I am radiant with good health.

DAY 15

You are midway through the 30-day program. Today, revisit Step 5 and look at my examples of self-love on page 72. How many can you check off affirmatively? For example, are you nourishing yourself with body-honoring foods? Are you avoiding self-criticism? Are you doing moving meditations? Congratulate yourself on the checkpoints you're living. Have the conversation with yourself and honor your progress. If there are some still to be worked on, write them down in your journal or *Just 10 Workbook*. Flip a few pages over and ask yourself the loving questions that will help you. Remember: If you can control the questions you ask yourself, you can begin to consciously change the way you feel about yourself, love yourself more, and ultimately change your circumstances. So ask—and answer—the questions that lead to a positive, productive, and action-oriented plan.

DAILY AFFIRMATION: Each step I take toward my dreams adds another harmonizing thread in the tapestry of my life. To live a consistently healthy, happy life, my thoughts and actions are positive and confident.

DAY 16

Review techniques you've learned so far and apply them. Try something like stopping your thoughts. Suppose you get the urge to eat a few pints of ice cream. To bring that urge under control, stop yourself and ask whether gorging on ice cream is a good way to honor your body. Thought-stopping is not a new psychological tool but it is a practical way to keep from getting stuck on those counterproductive thoughts. Today, list in your journal or *Just 10 Workbook* all the techniques that work for you, or that you think might work. Be open to success and your own blossoming health.

DAILY AFFIRMATION: I control my urges by focusing on thoughts that serve me and honor my body.

DAY 17

Take a lesson from competitive athletes. Start visualizing your new body. The toned muscles you'll have. The energy you'll feel. The smaller sizes you'll wear. See the "new you" entering a room with confidence and style. Trace your hands over your body as you step out of the shower and imagine how loved you are today. Nurture vivid images of yourself in which you are well and strong.

DAILY AFFIRMATION: I guide my thinking onto positive paths. Inspired thoughts enliven me and make my dreams real. I find comfort in my own evolution.

DAY 18

The most successfully completed projects are done a bit at a time. A building is constructed brick by brick. A race is won stride by stride. And a picture is painted stroke by stroke. In the same way, it's helpful to make daily manageable resolutions, rather than to set and focus on a far-off goal (which is why *Just 10* targets the first 10 pounds of your weight only). If all you do is concentrate on what you need to do today, achieving your goal is a cinch. Today, resolve to do just two things. Some examples of daily fitness resolutions might be:

- Reduce my intake of sugary or fatty foods.
- Eat two extra servings of vegetables.
- Increase my daily activity by 10 minutes.
- Play an active game with my kids.
- Learn a new form of exercise.

Continue to do this most days of the week. Before long, you'll be sliding into your skinny jeans or buckling your belt tighter.

DAILY AFFIRMATION: Today I make healthy new choices. And, I do the same tomorrow. Small changes build success.

DAY 19

Getting fit doesn't always come naturally—you probably know that from previous attempts to lose weight. But it can come supernaturally, if you connect to higher-source thinking that can give you the staying power you need. Ask your higher source to give you the strength to break destructive habits.

DAILY AFFIRMATION: I am in tune with the miracle-working power of God in my life; and I am grateful, happy, and optimistic.

DAY 20

Do you spend a lot of time in your car? Use this time to enrich yourself spiritually and emotionally. Today, listen to inspiring music or an audio book on your car stereo; read if you're taking public transportation; or if your day is filled with noisy kids or you work in a disruptive atmosphere, simply bask in the relative silence of your commute.

DAILY AFFIRMATION: I invite peace, joy, harmony, and God into my life wherever I am.

DAY 21

When faced with a good choice or a bad one, remember that the state of your life is the result of the choices you make—and the actions you take—in every moment. Remember how important our questions are, so ask yourself, *How can I best manage myself in this situation?* I think I know the correct answer. Do you?

DAILY AFFIRMATION: I make choices each day that determine the content and the outcome of my day.

DAY 22

At birth we're given the priceless gift of breath. Breathing keeps our body refreshed and renewed so that every part can function smoothly. It plays a vital role in keeping us whole and well. If something troubles you today, you can get instant relief with some simple deep breathing. Take 10 deep breaths through your nose with your mouth closed, and breathe out through your mouth. Breathe into your belly, not simply your lungs. Deep breathing slows your heart rate. Focusing on your breathing brings your awareness to how your body is feeling. Today, remember to give thanks to your higher source for clean, fresh air to breathe. Bless your body with the thought that every breath you take renews and revitalizes you.

DAILY AFFIRMATION: I use my breath to restore myself. I breathe in the positive and exhale the negative.

DAY 23

Many Bible verses start out with the phrase, "It came to pass." Not until I was older, wiser, and whole did I realize that this innocuous phrase has a subtle, extremely meaningful inference. There are times in life when you feel so hurt and frustrated that you're sure the pain will never pass. But it does, sometimes because of your efforts or sometimes because of the passage of time; but the problem always goes away. Reflect on any pain in your life right now with this in mind. The pain did not come into your life to stay; it came to pass. Accept it, but accept it as an experience that is just passing through. Something better is on the way.

DAILY AFFIRMATION: In the face of this challenge, I accept the reality of this situation, but not its permanence. It came to pass; it didn't come to stay.

DAY 24

Today, do a quick inventory of the people in your life. Who is in your corner and who is not? Keep yourself surrounded with positive, loving people, especially those who support your weight-loss efforts. If you are around negative people, you can't help but be influenced by them. This is why I believe so strongly in support groups, where there are people who have learned to deal with similar problems.

DAILY AFFIRMATION: I think of all the people who might appreciate my patience, gentleness, understanding, generosity, and more. My higher source has given me these gifts, and I am blessed as I celebrate them and pass them on to others.

DAY 25

Today, experience what it's like to put you first. Our natural inclination is to put ourselves on the back burner. We live in a time where it's virtuous to be a martyr, doing things out of duty rather than desire. We take on too many tasks because of a false assumption that we have more control over our lives if we do everything ourselves. We want to avoid saying "no" and looking like the bad guy. We don't want to be seen as selfish. Where does all this end? With feeling worn out and being overly reactive. I'm asking you to be selfish. No, I'm demanding that you be selfish so that you don't resort to self-destructive behaviors. Ask yourself, *Where am I in all of this?* Whether it's getting a long overdue checkup or going to the gym, you have to make yourself a priority again. Take good care of your emotional, physical, and spiritual well-being, so you can be there for others in a much healthier way.

DAILY AFFIRMATION: The time has come for me to *put myself first.* I follow through and do something special and important for myself today.

DAY 26

Use the power of touch to establish a more intimate connection between your mind and your body. In the shower or bath, massage soap or gel all over, focusing on the sensation of your own touch. Or before bed, apply body lotion, massaging it into your skin. Focus on a part of your body you don't like. After a few sessions of doing this exercise, you'll begin thinking more positively about that body part. Rub your temples, fingers, head, and toes. Give your "problem parts" more care than usual and your attitude toward them will change.

DAILY AFFIRMATION: My body is a beautiful temple, and I love it unconditionally.

DAY 27

Focus on the positive feedback you get from others. What prompts it? Is it your appearance? Your thoughtfulness? Your friendliness? Do more of the things that earn you praise, and bask in the way it makes you feel. Say "thank you" whenever people compliment you. Choose to believe the compliments people give you.

DAILY AFFIRMATION: I open my heart today, and I'm blessed by all that's around me. I build self-esteem as I practice estimable acts.

DAY 28

When I was a kid, I prayed to wheedle things out of God. I prayed for a dog. A baseball glove. A good grade on a math test and a shorter piano practice session. But I started feeling funny about praying to get things I wanted. I didn't know if that was right, or if I was even praying correctly. I asked my dad, who is a pastor, how to pray, and he replied that prayer isn't some magical chant or highly formalized recitation. Prayer, he said, is simply a conversation with a friend. When you call your friend on the phone, usually you'll say, "Hi, Jacki. How are you?" You start the same with God: "Hi, God. How are you?" And like any conversation between friends, it should be frank, honest, and open. "Pour out your heart," he told me. "Ask questions, request guidance, and share frustrations." So that's what I did, and that's what I do now. I discovered that God can be closer to us than even our closest friend. God longs to get involved with our lives and problems. The conversations bring me peace. Prayer is different for everyone; my advice for today is to harness its power to realign your attitudes toward life. No prayer ever goes unanswered.

DAILY AFFIRMATION: When trouble hits, I have peace. I ask for divine guidance in every activity today, and peace is mine.

DAY 29

Today build on your successes of the last few weeks. Acknowledge what you've accomplished and the ways you've changed. How much weight have you lost? How much more energy do you have? Are you less stressed or more at peace with yourself? What are you really excited about? Make a list of 10 things you feel good about.

DAILY AFFIRMATION: How far I have come! I keep moving forward, doing what I need to do, with success.

DAY 30

Make a plan to reward yourself and celebrate your successes. Rewards are great motivators. Today, decide what your reward will be. But first, a few rules: (1) Your reward should be a true treat— something you don't do for yourself often; (2) the reward should make you feel physically attractive, emotionally uplifted, spiritually inspired, just plain fun—or all of the above; (3) your reward should never tempt you to backslide. For instance, if you've lost those 10 pounds, resist rewarding yourself with a box of chocolate. Appropriate rewards give you the power to push on!

DAILY AFFIRMATION: I love this journey I'm on, and I celebrate my accomplishments and my life with joy, gratitude, and enthusiasm.

Living these steps and following this 30-day plan—all the things you can do to get and stay slim and healthy—will really make a big difference in achieving your fabulous new self. The 10 steps are a lifelong way of living; and while I've added whole grains now that I'm in the maintenance phase, I challenge you to not cheat on your food plan. Pledge to stick with the *Just 10* program without negotiation or delay. All you've got to lose is 10 pounds . . . for now! And the upside of what you'll gain is brilliant: A new understanding of food. A new perspective on exercise. A better sense of what motivates food cravings, along with know-how about what to do when they hit. Loving connections with your social circle and your spiritual self. All that and more.

I have witnessed the power of these steps to transform so many people, in so many ways, even in my own family.

I offer these steps as a gift to you. Make them part of your life.

Here's to seeing less of you, if you know what I mean.

The Love-Centered Diet Food Plan

Using these menus can make things easier for you, especially as you begin the plan. They include many recipes, which you may try if you wish. Let the menus guide you, but don't allow them to restrict you. If you like the same breakfast every day, that's fine—go ahead and enjoy something like the Berry Smoothie every morning, or eggs and fruit. If you don't like some of the food choices, don't force yourself to eat them. Substitute something else—another similar food or a different recipe—using the food lists and the Love-Centered Diet blueprint. But if a particular food is not on the plan, don't eat it. When in doubt, leave it out.

When you follow this plan, you're adjusting your body and appetite to what is best for your health and well-being. In the past, you've probably done the reverse—adjusting your intake of food to the demands of your appetite and emotions, with predictably chaotic results. Using this food plan and the eating-style strategies in Step 1, you can be more in touch with how your body feels and what it really needs. You'll find that nourishing, body-honoring foods are more satisfying than the vast quantities of empty calories you used to eat.

The Love-Centered Diet Menus

DAY 1

BREAKFAST
Berry Smoothie (see page 200)

LUNCH
Grilled boneless, skinless
   chicken breast atop 1 cup
   greens or 1 cup cut raw
   fibrous vegetables
½ cup baked sweet potato with
   1 tablespoon butter or olive oil
1 serving fruit

DINNER
Sea Bass in Parchment
(see page 202)

SNACKS
1 serving fruit

DAY 2

BREAKFAST
2 large eggs, scrambled
1 cup fresh berries
¼ cup low-fat yogurt

LUNCH
Pork chop, grilled
Turnips and Chard
  (see page 204)
1 serving fruit

DINNER
Roast beef tenderloin (make
  enough for two meals)
1 cup greens with 2 tablespoons dressing or olive oil
Cauliflower "Mashed Potatoes"
  (see page 215)

SNACKS
1 serving fruit

DAY 3

BREAKFAST
Yogurt Parfait (see page 214)

LUNCH
Leftover beef tenderloin
½ cup steamed peas
Heirloom Tomato Salad
  (see page 210)
1 serving fruit

DINNER
*Tempeh with Baby Bok Choy
and Mung Bean Sprouts*
  (see page 218)

SNACKS
1 serving fruit

DAY 4

BREAKFAST
Summer Frittata (see page 213)
1 fresh orange

LUNCH
Tuna fish (flaked fresh or
  canned albacore in water)
  served on 1 cup greens with
  1 tablespoon of salad dressing
  or olive oil

DINNER
Grilled chicken breast
1 cup raw or steamed carrots
1 cup greens or 1 cup cut raw
  fibrous vegetables with
  2 tablespoons dressing or
  olive oil

SNACKS
1 serving fruit

DAY 5

BREAKFAST
1¼ cup low-fat Greek-style
yogurt
*Fresh Figs and Raspberries
Drizzled with Honey*
(see page 215)

LUNCH
Ham, lean
Steamed green beans
1 cup greens or 1 cup cut raw
fibrous vegetables with 1 tablespoon dressing or olive oil
1 serving fruit

DINNER
Roasted turkey breast
(make enough for two meals)
1 cup steamed peas
Cauliflower "Mashed Potatoes"
(see page 215)

SNACKS
1 serving fruit

DAY 6

BREAKFAST
Fruit shake: Blend together
1¼ cup low-fat milk and 1 cup
frozen unsweetened berries
(and ice if desired)

LUNCH
Leftover roast turkey
Long Bean Salad (see page 211)
1 cup greens or 1 cup cut
raw fibrous vegetables with
1 tablespoon dressing or
olive oil
Broiled Pears (see page 214)

DINNER
*Roasted Cherry Tomatoes with
Free-Range Eggs* (see page 212)
1 cup greens or 1 cup cut
raw fibrous vegetables with
2 tablespoons salad dressing
or olive oil
1 serving fruit

SNACKS
1 serving fruit

DAY 7

BREAKFAST
Blue and Peach (see page 210)
1¼ cup low-fat Greek-style
  yogurt

LUNCH
Grilled chicken atop 1 cup
  greens
1 cup steamed eggplant
  drizzled with 1 tablespoon
  sesame oil
1 serving fruit

DINNER
Sesame Shrimp over Watercress
  (see page 208)
*Butternut Squash and Baby
  Arugula Salad* (see page 214)

SNACKS
1 serving fruit

DAY 8

BREAKFAST
2 large scrambled or poached
  eggs
1 sliced peach or other seasonal
  fruit
½ cup low-fat cottage cheese

LUNCH
*Red Chili Tofu with Summer
  Squash* (see page 211)
1 cup greens or 1 cup cut raw
  fibrous vegetables with
  1 tablespoon dressing or
  olive oil
1 serving fruit

DINNER
Sage and Garlic Pork
  (see page 217)
½ cup roasted winter squash
1 cup raw broccoli and
  cauliflower mix drizzled with
  2 tablespoons sesame oil

SNACKS
1 serving fruit

DAY 9

BREAKFAST
Berry Smoothie (see page 200)

LUNCH
Soft Scrambled Eggs with Crumbled Feta, Wilted Spinach, and Baby Tomatoes
(see page 217)
1 serving fruit

DINNER
Grilled salmon
Salad Greens with Miso-Ginger Dressing (see page 203)
Asparagus with Lemon
(see page 205)

SNACKS
1 serving fruit

DAY 10

BREAKFAST
Turkey bacon
½ grapefruit
¼ cup low-fat Greek-style yogurt

LUNCH
Ham, lean
1 cup steamed green beans
½ cup roasted winter squash drizzled with 1 tablespoon olive oil
1 serving fruit

DINNER
Ahi Tuna and Scallions
(see page 209)
Raw Kale Salad (see page 201)
½ cup baked sweet potato with 2 tablespoons butter

SNACKS
1 serving fruit

DAY 11

BREAKFAST
Asparagus, Leek, and Herb Tofu
Scramble (see page 205)
1 cup fresh berries

LUNCH
Rosemary Chicken (see page 216)
Cauliflower "Mashed Potatoes"
(see page 215)
1 cup greens or 1 cup cut
raw fibrous vegetables with
1 tablespoon salad dressing
or olive oil
1 serving fruit

DINNER
Cumin-Crusted Spring Lamb
with Yogurt-Mint Sauce
(see page 207)
½ cup steamed peas
1 cup greens or 1 cup cut
raw fibrous vegetables with
2 tablespoons salad dressing
or olive oil

SNACKS
1 serving fruit

DAY 12

BREAKFAST
Yogurt Parfait (see page 214)

LUNCH
Tofu and Seaweed Soup
(see page 203)
1 cup roasted carrots with
1 tablespoon salad dressing
or olive oil
1 serving fruit

DINNER
Sesame Shrimp Over Watercress
(see page 208)
½ cup steamed peas
1 cup greens or 1 cup cut
raw fibrous vegetables with
2 tablespoons salad dressing
or olive oil

SNACKS
1 serving fruit

DAY 13

BREAKFAST
2 large scrambled or poached
  eggs
1 cup fresh berries
¼ cup low-fat Greek-style
  yogurt

LUNCH
*Chicken and Mint Salad with
Yellow Bell Peppers*
(see page 206)
1 cup steamed eggplant
1 serving fruit

DINNER
Grilled sirloin steak
1 cup mashed parsnips
1 cup greens or 1 cup cut
  raw fibrous vegetables with
  2 tablespoons dressing or
  olive oil

SNACKS
1 serving fruit

DAY 14

BREAKFAST
Berry Smoothie (see page 200)

LUNCH
2 ounces cheddar cheese
  and 2 ounces lean ham
  served on 1 cup greens with
  1 tablespoon salad dressing
  or olive oil
½ cup roasted beets
1 serving fruit

DINNER
Peel-and-eat shrimp with
  cocktail sauce (make your
  own with lemon, crushed
  tomatoes, and horseradish)
1 cup steamed green beans
2 tomatoes and 1 cucumber,
  sliced, with 1 tablespoon
  salad dressing or olive oil

SNACKS
1 serving fruit

DAY 15

BREAKFAST
2 large scrambled or poached
  eggs
½ grapefruit
¼ cup low-fat cottage cheese

LUNCH
Grilled chicken atop 1 cup
  greens
½ cup sliced pickled beets
  drizzled with 1 tablespoon of
  salad dressing or olive oil
1 serving fruit

DINNER
*Wild-Caught Alaskan Salmon
with Asian Pesto and Wilted
Greens* (see page 208)
½ cup mashed cooked
  pumpkin with 2 tablespoons
  butter or olive oil

SNACKS
1 serving fruit

DAY 16

BREAKFAST
Berry Smoothie (see page 200)

LUNCH
Tuna atop 1 cup greens with
  1 tablespoon salad dressing or
  olive oil
1 serving fruit

DINNER
*Chicken Sausage with Turnips
and Winter Greens*
(see page 201)
½ roasted acorn squash with
  2 tablespoons butter or
  olive oil

SNACKS
1 serving fruit

DAY 17

BREAKFAST
2 large eggs, scrambled
1 sectioned apple
¼ cup low-fat cottage cheese

LUNCH
2 ounces cheese
*Cucumber Salad with Sesame-
Lemon Dressing* (see page 206)
1 serving fruit

DINNER
Roast beef tenderloin (make
enough for two meals)
1 cup greens or 1 cup cut
raw fibrous vegetables with
2 tablespoons salad dressing
or olive oil
Cauliflower "Mashed Potatoes"
(see page 215)

SNACKS
1 serving fruit

DAY 18

BREAKFAST
Yogurt Parfait (see page 214)

LUNCH
Leftover beef tenderloin
½ cup steamed peas
1 cup greens or 1 cup cut
raw fibrous vegetables with
1 tablespoon salad dressing
or olive oil
1 serving fruit

DINNER
Grilled Chicken with Basil
(see page 210)
½ cup cooked carrots
1 cup greens with 2 tablespoons salad dressing or
olive oil

SNACKS
1 serving fruit

DAY 19

BREAKFAST
Summer Frittata (see page 213)
1 fresh sliced peach or other
  seasonal fruit
¼ cup cottage cheese

LUNCH
Grilled chicken atop 1 cup
  greens with 1 tablespoon
  salad dressing or olive oil
½ cup sweet potato
1 serving fruit

DINNER
Grey Sole and Lacinato Kale
  (see page 216)
½ cup cooked carrots
1 cup greens with
  2 tablespoons salad
  dressing or olive oil

SNACKS
1 serving fruit

DAY 20

BREAKFAST
1¼ cup low-fat Greek-style
  yogurt
1 pear, sliced

LUNCH
2 ounces cheddar cheese and
  2 ounces lean ham served
  on 1 cup greens with
  1 tablespoon salad dressing
  or olive oil
1 serving fruit

DINNER
Roasted turkey breast
  (make enough for two meals)
½ cup steamed peas
Cauliflower "Mashed Potatoes"
  (see page 215)

SNACKS
1 serving fruit

DAY 21

BREAKFAST
Fruit shake: Blend together
1¼ cup low-fat milk and 1 cup
frozen unsweetened berries
(and ice if desired)

LUNCH
Leftover roast turkey
Broiled Pears (see page 214)
1 cup greens or a diced
cucumber, a tomato, and
a carrot with 1 tablespoon
salad dressing or olive oil

DINNER
Sage and Garlic Pork
(see page 217)
*Butternut Squash and Baby
Arugula Salad* (see page 214)
1 cup steamed broccoli

SNACKS
1 serving fruit

DAY 22

BREAKFAST
Warm Winter Fruit Sauté
(see page 204)
1 cup low-fat Greek-style
yogurt

LUNCH
Grilled or broiled shrimp
atop 1 cup greens with
1 tablespoon salad dressing
or olive oil
1 serving fruit

DINNER
Grilled sirloin steak
1 cup cooked carrots with
2 tablespoons butter or
olive oil
Cauliflower "Mashed Potatoes"
(see page 215)

SNACKS
1 serving fruit

DAY 23

BREAKFAST
2 large scrambled or poached
 eggs
1 sliced pear or other seasonal
 fruit
¼ cup low-fat cottage cheese

LUNCH
*Red Chili Tofu with Summer
 Squash* (see page 211)
1 cup greens or 1 cup cut raw
 fibrous vegetables
1 serving fruit

DINNER
Sage and Garlic Pork
 (see page 217)
½ cup roasted winter squash
1 cup greens or 1 cup cut
 raw fibrous vegetables with
 2 tablespoons salad dressing
 or olive oil

SNACKS
1 serving fruit

DAY 24

BREAKFAST
Berry Smoothie (see page 200)

LUNCH
*Seared Steak, Edamame, and
 Snow Pea Salad* (see page 212)
1 cup greens or 1 cup cut
 raw fibrous vegetables with
 1 tablespoon salad dressing
 or olive oil
1 serving fruit

DINNER
Grilled salmon
½ cup roasted beets
Long Bean Salad (see page 211)

SNACKS
1 serving fruit

DAY 25

BREAKFAST
Turkey bacon
1 cup fresh berries
¼ cup low-fat Greek-style
 yogurt

LUNCH
Ham, lean
Shaved Zucchini Salad
 (see page 213)
½ cup baked sweet potato
1 serving fruit

DINNER
Ahi Tuna and Scallions
 (see page 209)
Lemon Spring Vegetables
 (see page 207)
½ cup roasted winter squash

SNACKS
1 serving fruit

DAY 26

BREAKFAST
*Asparagus, Leek, and Herb Tofu
 Scramble* (see page 205)
1 fresh orange

LUNCH
2 ounces cheddar cheese and
 2 ounces lean ham atop 1 cup
 greens with 1 tablespoon
 salad dressing or olive oil
½ cup roasted beets
1 serving fruit

DINNER
*Cumin-Crusted Spring Lamb
 with Yogurt-Mint Sauce*
 (see page 207)
½ cup roasted winter squash
1 cup greens or 1 cup cut
 raw fibrous vegetables with
 2 tablespoons salad dressing
 or olive oil

SNACKS
1 serving fruit

DAY 27

BREAKFAST
Yogurt Parfait (see page 214)

LUNCH
Grilled chicken atop 1 cup
greens or 1 cut carrot, 1 cut
cucumber, and 1 cut tomato
with 1 tablespoon salad
dressing or olive oil
1 serving fruit

DINNER
Sesame Shrimp over Watercress
(see page 208)
½ cup steamed peas
1 cup greens with
2 tablespoons salad
dressing or olive oil

SNACKS
Fresh fruit

DAY 28

BREAKFAST
2 large scrambled or poached
eggs
1 cup fresh berries
¼ cup low-fat Greek-style
yogurt

LUNCH
*Chicken and Mint Salad with
Yellow Bell Peppers*
(see page 206)
½ cup sweet potato drizzled
with 1 tablespoon butter or
olive oil
1 serving fruit

DINNER
Grilled sirloin steak
1 cup mashed parsnips
Celery Root Salad (see page
215) with *White Balsamic
Vinaigrette* (see page 218)

SNACKS
1 serving fruit

DAY 29

BREAKFAST
Berry Smoothie (see page 200)

LUNCH
Seared Steak, Edamame, and Snow Pea Salad (see page 212)
1 cup greens or 1 cup cut raw fibrous vegetables with 1 tablespoon salad dressing or olive oil
1 serving fruit

DINNER
Peel-and-eat shrimp with cocktail sauce (homemade with lemon, crushed tomatoes, spices, and horseradish)
Steamed green beans
Frisée and Fennel Salad (see page 216) with *White Balsamic Vinaigrette* (see page 218)

SNACKS
1 serving fruit

DAY 30

BREAKFAST
2 large scrambled or poached eggs
1 cup fresh berries
¼ cup low-fat Greek-style yogurt

LUNCH
Grilled chicken atop 1 cup greens
½ cup sliced pickled beets drizzled with 2 tablespoons of salad dressing or olive oil
1 serving fruit

DINNER
Wild-Caught Alaskan Salmon with Asian Pesto and Wilted Greens (see page 208)
½ cup baked pumpkin drizzled with 2 tablespoons butter or olive oil

SNACKS
1 serving fruit

The Love-Centered Diet Recipes

My friend Lisa Roberts-Lehan, who cooked up the menus and recipes in *Just 10*, is an Oxford-educated archaeologist who attended the French Culinary Institute to become a classically trained chef. She wanted to help kids and adults live better following her own life-saving changes around food. "I was dying from food, and it was a lifelong affair that had left me emotionally brittle and hurting." Lisa's cooking on all burners now; and I love how she's helping others reframe their relationship with food through amazingly tantalizing, tasty, self-loving recipes. You can find more of her amazing recipes online at *Just10Diet.com*.

The recipes are organized seasonally. It's preferable to eat fruits and vegetables in season, because they hold the most nutrition and flavor. I realize this is not always possible, however, and most grocery stores supply the majority of these foods year-round.

Each recipe yields only one serving, so if you're cooking for other people in addition to yourself, simply multiply each amount by the number of people who will be eating. Enjoy!

WINTER RECIPES

BERRY SMOOTHIE

1¼ cup cold nonfat milk (or unsweetened soy, nut,
   or rice milk)
1 cup fresh or frozen strawberries or blueberries
1 teaspoon alcohol-free vanilla extract

In a blender, combine all of the ingredients and blend on high until smooth.

CHICKEN SAUSAGE WITH TURNIPS AND WINTER GREENS

3 teaspoons extra-virgin olive oil, divided
4 ounces organic chicken sausage, cut into ¼-inch slices
1 teaspoon shallot, minced
1 clove garlic, minced
1 cup Swiss chard, collards, kale, or turnip greens, thinly
    sliced, tough stems removed
3 cups salted water (3 cups water and
    ½ teaspoon salt)
1 turnip, peeled and chopped into ¼-inch cubes
Sea salt and freshly ground black pepper, to taste

In a sauté pan over medium heat, warm 2 teaspoons of oil. Add sausage and cook 4 to 5 minutes, or until brown on both sides. Transfer to a plate and set aside. In the same sauté pan, over medium-low heat, use remaining 1 teaspoon oil to cook shallot. Add garlic and sauté another 15 seconds, or until fragrant. Add the greens and sauté until tender.

In medium sauce pan, bring 3 cups salted water to a boil and blanch turnips until tender. Season with salt and pepper. Add turnips and warm with the greens. To serve, arrange the vegetables and top with the sausage.

RAW KALE SALAD

2 cups curly kale, tough stems removed
1½ tablespoons extra-virgin olive oil
1 teaspoon Bragg Liquid Aminos
1 teaspoon red pepper flakes
⅛ teaspoon cayenne
Juice of ½ lemon

In a large bowl, tear the kale leaves into bite-size pieces. Add the remaining ingredients and toss with your hands to thoroughly coat the leaves. Adjust seasoning to taste.

SEA BASS IN PARCHMENT

One 4-ounce sea bass fillet (halibut or Arctic char can
   be substituted)
1 teaspoon extra-virgin olive oil
1 teaspoon fresh thyme, chopped
½ tablespoon butter
1 carrot, trimmed, peeled, and cut in ⅛-inch matchsticks
1 rib celery, cut into ⅛-inch matchsticks
1 leek, white part only, cut into ⅛-inch matchsticks
Juice of ½ lemon
1 sprig fresh thyme
Sea salt and freshly ground black pepper, to taste
1 egg white, lightly beaten
½ teaspoon vegetable oil

Preheat the oven to 450° F. Lightly brush the fillet with 1 teaspoon olive oil and sprinkle with thyme. Place on a plate, cover, and refrigerate.

In a sauté pan over medium heat, melt the butter and add the carrots and celery. Add 2 tablespoons water and gently sauté for about 5 minutes. Add the leeks and cook until the vegetables are tender, another 2 to 3 minutes. Remove from heat and set aside.

Cut a piece of parchment paper to measure about 12 by 18 inches. Place the fish in the middle of the paper, garnish with a squeeze of lemon, and top with vegetables and sprig of thyme. Season with a sprinkling of salt and pepper. To seal, fold over the long sides of the parchment twice, and then roll in the short sides. Brush with egg white to seal. Lightly coat top of the packet with ½ teaspoon vegetable oil. Place the packet on a baking sheet and bake for about 8 minutes, or until the packets puff up. Remove from oven and serve.

SALAD GREENS WITH MISO-GINGER DRESSING

1 cup salad greens
¼ cup shredded daikon
¼ cup shredded carrots
1 scallion, white part only, thinly sliced
Toasted sesame seeds, for garnish

MISO-GINGER DRESSING
2 tablespoons water, plus more to taste
½ tablespoon white (*shiro*) miso
1 tablespoon tahini
¼ teaspoon fresh ginger, finely grated
¼ teaspoon agave nectar
1 teaspoon lemon juice
Freshly ground black pepper, to taste
Sea salt or Bragg Liquid Aminos, to taste

In a bowl, whisk all of the dressing ingredients together. Set aside. Arrange the salad greens, daikon, and carrots on a plate and drizzle with dressing. Garnish with sesame seeds.

TOFU AND SEAWEED SOUP

3 cups low-sodium vegetable or chicken broth
Pinch garlic powder
1 teaspoon Bragg Liquid Aminos or low-sodium soy sauce
1 cup thinly sliced Napa cabbage
4 ounces tofu, diced
1 sheet nori, cut into matchsticks, for garnish

Heat the broth over medium-high heat, season with garlic powder and Bragg Liquid Aminos or low-sodium soy sauce. When the broth is heated, add the cabbage and tofu. Serve in a bowl and garnish with nori.

TURNIPS AND CHARD

3 cups salted water (3 cups water and
  ½ teaspoon salt)
1 turnip, peeled and chopped into small dice
1 clove garlic, minced
1 teaspoon minced shallot
1 teaspoon extra-virgin olive oil
1 cup Swiss chard, thinly sliced, tough stems removed
Sea salt and freshly ground black pepper, to taste

In a medium saucepan, bring approximately 3 cups of salted water
to a boil, then blanch the turnips until tender.

In a sauté pan, sweat shallots in oil over medium-low heat. Add
the garlic and sweat another 15 seconds, or until fragrant. Add the
greens and sauté until tender. Season with salt and pepper. Add the
turnips and warm with the greens. Serve.

WARM WINTER FRUIT SAUTÉ

¼ teaspoon coconut oil
1 cup sliced apples or pears (or a combination of the two)
Pinch cinnamon
Pinch nutmeg

In a sauté pan over medium heat, gently cook the coconut oil, apples,
and pears for 2 to 3 minutes. Add 1 to 2 tablespoons of water, cinnamon,
and nutmeg, and stir to coat. Simmer for another 5 minutes. If the
juice evaporates before dish is done, add more water. Serve.

SPRING RECIPES

ASPARAGUS, LEEK, AND HERB TOFU SCRAMBLE

8 ounces low-fat tofu, silken or firm
1 teaspoon extra-virgin olive oil
½ cup asparagus, trimmed and chopped into 2-inch lengths
¼ cup chopped leeks, white parts only
1 teaspoon Bragg Liquid Aminos
¼ teaspoon garam masala
1 teaspoon fresh parsley, chopped

Crumble the tofu in a bowl. In a sauté pan over medium heat, warm the olive oil and add the asparagus, leeks, and Bragg Liquid Aminos, sautéing for 3 to 4 minutes. Add the tofu and garam masala, stirring frequently for 5 to 7 minutes. Sprinkle with parsley and serve.

ASPARAGUS WITH LEMON

¼ pound asparagus, trimmed
Juice of ¼ lemon
1 teaspoon grated lemon zest (optional)
Sea salt and freshly ground black pepper, to taste

Steam asparagus and simply season with a squeeze of lemon, a sprinkling of lemon zest, salt, and pepper.

CHICKEN AND MINT SALAD WITH YELLOW BELL PEPPERS

4 ounces boneless, skinless chicken breast
3 tablespoons extra-virgin olive oil, divided
Sea salt and freshly ground black pepper or cayenne
   pepper, to taste
1 yellow bell pepper, sliced
Juice of ½ lemon
¼ cup mint leaves
¼ cup cilantro leaves
Frisée, arugula, or other baby salad greens
Cooking spray

Preheat the oven to 375°F. Coat the chicken in 1 tablespoon of olive oil and season with salt and pepper. (If you like heat, substitute the black pepper with cayenne.) Place the chicken on a foil-lined baking sheet coated with cooking spray and bake for 25 to 30 minutes on the center rack, or until juices run clear.

In sauté pan over medium heat, warm a tablespoon of olive oil and sauté the yellow peppers for about 5 minutes. Season to taste.

To make the dressing, whisk the juice of half a lemon with 1 tablespoon of olive oil in a nonreactive bowl and season to taste.

Once the chicken is done, allow to rest for 5 minutes before slicing. Combine chicken with the mint, cilantro, bell peppers, and salad greens. Toss with lemon juice and olive-oil dressing. Adjust seasonings and serve.

CUCUMBER SALAD WITH SESAME-LEMON DRESSING

1 seedless cucumber, shaved into ribbons
1 tablespoon sesame oil
Juice of ½ lemon
½ tablespoon sesame seeds
Sea salt
Pinch of red pepper flakes

In a bowl, toss the ingredients and serve.

CUMIN-CRUSTED SPRING LAMB WITH YOGURT-MINT SAUCE

One 4-ounce lamb fillet
¼ teaspoon ground cumin or crushed cumin seeds
1 teaspoon extra-virgin olive oil
Sea salt and freshly ground black pepper, to taste
½ cucumber, thinly sliced
¼ cup mint leaves
1 cup baby arugula leaves

YOGURT-MINT SAUCE:
⅛ cup plain, nonfat yogurt
1 teaspoon lemon juice
1 teaspoon fresh mint, finely chopped

To make the yogurt sauce, combine the yogurt, lemon juice, and mint in a nonreactive bowl and set aside.

Place the lamb, cumin, oil, salt, and pepper in a bowl and thoroughly coat. In a nonstick sauté pan over medium heat, cook the lamb 2 to 3 minutes on each side. Let rest 5 minutes before slicing. Serve lamb over cucumber, mint leaves, and baby arugula. Drizzle with yogurt-mint sauce.

LEMON SPRING VEGETABLES

4 cups salted water (4 cups water with ½ teaspoon salt)
½ cup green beans, trimmed and chopped
½ cup sugar snap peas, trimmed
⅛ cup lemon juice
½ tablespoon finely grated lemon zest
1 tablespoon extra-virgin olive oil
1 tablespoon fresh flat-leaf parsley leaves
Sea salt and freshly ground black pepper, to taste

Bring a saucepan of salted water to a boil and cook the green beans and sugar snap peas for 1 minute. Drain and immediately shock in ice water. In a bowl, toss beans and peas with the lemon juice, zest, olive oil, parsley, salt, and pepper. Serve.

SESAME SHRIMP OVER WATERCRESS

1 pinch Chinese five-spice
3 tablespoons sesame seeds
1 egg white, lightly beaten
4 ounces shrimp, peeled and deveined
1 teaspoon sesame oil
1 cup watercress, washed and trimmed
½ cucumber, thinly sliced

LIME VINAIGRETTE:
3 tablespoons lime juice
1 tablespoon sesame oil
½ teaspoon agave nectar
½ teaspoon Bragg Liquid Aminos or low-sodium soy sauce

To make the vinaigrette, whisk together all of the ingredients in a small bowl. Set aside.

To make the shrimp, place the five-spice and sesame seeds in a bowl and thoroughly combine. Set aside. In another bowl, add the egg white and shrimp and toss to coat. Press the shrimp into the spice-and-sesame mixture. In a nonstick sauté pan over medium-high heat, heat 1 teaspoon sesame oil, add shrimp, and cook for about 1 minute each side, or until golden. Lightly coat the watercress and cucumbers with vinaigrette and top with the shrimp. Serve.

WILD-CAUGHT ALASKAN SALMON WITH ASIAN PESTO AND WILTED GREENS

PESTO:
1 tablespoon finely chopped fresh cilantro
1 tablespoon finely chopped fresh mint
1 tablespoon finely chopped fresh parsley
1 tablespoon fresh scallion
½ teaspoon freshly grated ginger
½ clove of garlic, minced
Juice of ½ lime
½ tablespoon sesame oil
½ teaspoon Bragg Liquid Aminos or low-sodium soy sauce

SALMON:

One 4-ounce salmon fillet, bones removed

Cooking spray

GREENS:

1 teaspoon sesame oil

¼ pound collards, baby bok choy, spinach, tatsoi, or other greens

¼ teaspoon garlic, minced

¼ teaspoon freshly grated ginger

2 or 3 tablespoons low-sodium vegetable broth or water

⅛ teaspoon Bragg Liquid Aminos or low-sodium soy sauce

Preheat the oven to 450°F. Place the pesto ingredients in a food processor and blend until smooth. Evenly coat the fish with pesto, reserving some for garnish after baking, and place in a baking dish coated with cooking spray. Bake for 8 minutes or until slightly undercooked. Meanwhile, in a nonstick pan, over medium-high heat, warm 1 teaspoon sesame oil and gently sauté the greens for about 3 minutes. Add the garlic, ginger, vegetable broth, and Bragg Liquid Aminos, sautéing another minute. Transfer greens to a plate and top with the salmon fillet and fresh pesto.

SUMMER RECIPES

AHI TUNA AND SCALLIONS

1 cup scallions cut into 1-inch pieces

1½ teaspoons extra-virgin olive oil, divided

½ teaspoon Bragg Liquid Aminos or low-sodium soy sauce

One 4-ounce ahi tuna fillet

1 teaspoon toasted black or white sesame seeds

Preheat broiler. In a large sauté pan over medium heat, heat ½ teaspoon olive oil and sauté the scallions. Set aside.

In a small bowl, mix together 1 teaspoon olive oil and Bragg Liquid Aminos. Add the tuna and toss to coat. Place the fish on a foil-lined baking sheet and broil for 3 to 5 minutes on each side. To serve, garnish the tuna with scallions and a sprinkling of sesame seeds.

BLUE AND PEACH

½ cup blueberries
½ cup sliced peaches

Toss to combine. Serve alone or over Greek-style yogurt.

GRILLED CHICKEN WITH BASIL

One 4-ounce boneless, skinless organic chicken breast
2 tablespoons fresh basil, chopped, plus extra for garnish
¼ teaspoon fresh garlic, minced
Sea salt and freshly ground black pepper, to taste
1 teaspoon extra-virgin olive oil

In a bowl, combine the chicken, basil, garlic, salt and pepper, and olive oil. Cover and marinate in the refrigerator for 10 minutes. Remove chicken from the marinade and grill or broil. Grill about 7 minutes on each side, or until juices run clear. If broiling, set rack about 5 inches from heat source and cook 4 to 5 minutes each side, or until juices run clear. Garnish with extra herbs and serve.

HEIRLOOM TOMATO SALAD

1 cup heirloom tomatoes, sliced
2 teaspoons extra-virgin olive oil
Sea salt and freshly ground black pepper, to taste
1 tablespoon fresh basil, tightly rolled and finely sliced

In a bowl, toss tomatoes, olive oil, salt, and pepper. Allow to marinate for 20 minutes. To serve, garnish with basil.

LONG BEAN SALAD

1 cup mixed long beans (green, purple, romano, yellow, or
   wax beans)
Juice of ½ lemon
Sea salt and freshly ground black pepper, to taste

Blanch the beans in boiling water for 1 minute. Drain and quickly
shock in ice-cold water. Squeeze with lemon, season, and serve.

RED CHILI TOFU WITH SUMMER SQUASH

2 tablespoons lemon juice
1 teaspoon sesame oil
½ teaspoon Bragg Liquid Aminos
½ teaspoon red chili flakes
1 clove garlic, minced
½ teaspoon agave nectar
Sea salt and freshly ground black pepper, to taste
One 4-ounce block low-fat firm or extra-firm tofu, cut into
   cubes or ¼-inch slices
1 cup summer squash, sliced
1 scallion, thinly sliced

In a bowl, combine lemon juice, sesame oil, Bragg Liquid Aminos,
chili flakes, garlic, agave, salt, and pepper. Add the tofu and summer
squash, and toss to coat. Allow to marinate for at least 10 minutes.
In a sauté pan over medium heat, cook the squash for about 4 to 5
minutes. Transfer to a bowl and set aside. Add the tofu slices to the
pan and cook 4 to 5 minutes each side. To serve, drizzle the plated
tofu and squash with the chili marinade and garnish with scallions.

ROASTED CHERRY TOMATOES WITH FREE-RANGE EGGS

4 cherry tomatoes
1 teaspoon extra-virgin olive oil
Sea salt and freshly ground pepper, to taste
Cooking spray
2 large organic free-range eggs

Preheat the oven to 400°F. Place the tomatoes in a baking dish, drizzle with oil, and sprinkle with salt and pepper. Roast for 20 to 25 minutes, or until soft. Set aside. Coat large nonstick pan with cooking spray and warm over medium-high heat. Crack the eggs into the pan and cook for 3 to 4 minutes or until the yolks are just set. Serve with the tomatoes and season with sea salt and freshly ground black pepper.

SEARED STEAK, EDAMAME, AND SNOW PEA SALAD

4 ounces grass-fed top round steak, ¾-inch thick, trimmed
   of fat
⅛ teaspoon sea salt
¼ teaspoon freshly ground black pepper
Cooking spray
1 cup snow peas, thawed and sliced into matchsticks
¼ cup edamame, shelled
1 tablespoon lime juice
1 tablespoon extra-virgin olive oil, divided
1 long red chili, finely chopped
2 cups mixed Asian greens or salad greens
1 cucumber, sliced
⅛ cup cilantro leaves

Season steak with salt and pepper. In a nonstick sauté pan over medium heat, coated with cooking spray, cook the steak for 4 minutes per side for medium-rare. Set aside and let rest for at least 5 minutes before slicing. Return pan to heat and gently sauté snow peas and edamame for 1 to 2 minutes, until warmed.

To make the dressing, whisk together the lime juice, olive oil, and the red chili.

Combine greens, cucumber, snow peas, edamame, cilantro, and dressing in a large bowl. Toss to coat. Plate and top with the steak. Serve.

SHAVED ZUCCHINI SALAD

1 zucchini, trimmed
2 tablespoons extra-virgin olive oil
Juice of ½ lemon
½ teaspoon red pepper flakes (optional)
Sea salt

With a vegetable peeler, shave the zucchini from top to bottom. Place zucchini ribbons in a bowl and toss with remaining ingredients. Serve.

SUMMER FRITTATA

Cooking spray
¼ cup red, yellow, or orange bell pepper, diced
¼ cup zucchini, diced
2 large eggs
Pinch of sea salt
⅛ teaspoon freshly ground black pepper
1 tablespoon reduced-fat cheese
¼ cup tomatoes, chopped
1 tablespoon fresh basil leaves, tightly rolled and
    thinly sliced

In a nonstick sauté pan coated with cooking spray over medium-high heat, cook pepper and zucchini about 7 minutes, or until tender. In a medium bowl, whisk together eggs, salt, and pepper. Pour egg mixture over hot vegetables in pan; add cheese and stir gently to combine. Reduce heat to medium-low. Cook without stirring about 5 minutes, or until eggs are set on bottom. Garnish with tomatoes and basil.

YOGURT PARFAIT

1 cup nonfat Greek-style yogurt
1 cup mixed berries (raspberries, blueberries, blackberries,
    or strawberries)
Stevia to taste

In a tall parfait glass, alternate layers of yogurt and berries. Serve
and enjoy.

FALL RECIPES

BROILED PEARS

Cooking spray
1 pear, unpeeled, halved, cored, thinly sliced lengthwise
½ teaspoon extra-virgin coconut oil
Pinch cinnamon (optional)

Preheat broiler. Coat a baking sheet with cooking spray. Gently toss
pears with coconut oil. Arrange fruit in single layer on baking sheet.
Broil about 5 minutes, or until fruit is tender and edges begin to
brown. Sprinkle with optional cinnamon and serve. You can also
substitute apples for this recipe.

BUTTERNUT SQUASH AND BABY ARUGULA SALAD

Cooking spray
½ cup butternut squash, cut into cubes
¼ teaspoon fresh rosemary or sage, minced
1¼ teaspoon extra-virgin olive oil, divided
Sea salt and freshly ground black pepper, to taste
2 cups baby arugula or other salad greens
½ teaspoon balsamic vinegar

Preheat oven to 400°F. Coat a baking sheet with cooking spray
or line with parchment paper. In a bowl, toss squash with herbs,

¼ teaspoon of the olive oil, and salt and pepper. Spread in a single layer on the baking sheet and roast for about 30 minutes, or until tender and slightly browned. Flip squash halfway through cooking. Toss salad greens with 1 tablespoon olive oil and ½ teaspoon balsamic vinegar. Add butternut squash and toss. Serve.

CAULIFLOWER "MASHED POTATOES"

¼ head of cauliflower
¼ teaspoon garlic powder
1 tablespoon extra-virgin olive oil
1 to 3 tablespoons vegetable broth
Sea salt and freshly ground black pepper, to taste

Steam cauliflower with garlic powder. In a food processor, add cauliflower, olive oil, and vegetable broth, and pulse until as smooth as "mashed potatoes." Season with salt and pepper and serve.

CELERY ROOT SALAD

1 cup celery root (celeriac), peeled and cut into ⅛-inch matchsticks
White Balsamic Vinaigrette (see page 218)

In a bowl, toss celery root with White Balsamic Vinaigrette.

FRESH FIGS AND RASPBERRIES DRIZZLED WITH HONEY

½ cup fresh figs, halved or quartered
½ cup fresh raspberries
1 teaspoon 100% pure honey

Arrange figs and raspberries on a plate or in a bowl and drizzle with honey.

FRISÉE AND FENNEL SALAD

1 cup frisée lettuce, chopped
1 cup fennel, chopped or shaved
White Balsamic Vinaigrette (see page 218)

In a bowl, toss ingredients with White Balsamic Vinaigrette.

GREY SOLE AND LACINATO KALE

Cooking spray
One 4-ounce fillet of Grey or Dover sole
2 teaspoons extra-virgin olive oil, divided
Juice of ½ lemon
Sea salt and freshly ground black pepper, to taste
1 sprig fresh thyme
1 bunch lacinato (dinosaur or Tuscan) kale, thinly sliced,
    tough stems removed
1 clove garlic, minced

Preheat oven to 350°F. Coat an 8-by-11-inch piece of aluminum foil with cooking spray. Lay the fillet skin-side down on the foil and season with 1 teaspoon of the oil and the juice, salt, pepper, and thyme. Loosely seal the foil around the fish and place the package on a baking sheet. Bake for 10 minutes or until the fish is opaque and flakes easily.

In a sauté pan over medium heat, warm 1 teaspoon olive oil and sauté the garlic, stirring frequently, for about 15 seconds. Add the kale and 2 tablespoons of water. Continue to sauté until the water evaporates and the leaves are tender.

To serve, arrange the kale and top with the sole.

ROSEMARY CHICKEN

One 4-ounce boneless, skinless organic chicken breast
1 teaspoon extra-virgin olive oil
2 tablespoons fresh rosemary, chopped
¼ teaspoon fresh garlic, minced
Sea salt and freshly ground black pepper, to taste

In a bowl, combine the ingredients, cover, and marinate in the refrigerator for 10 minutes. Remove chicken from the marinade and grill or broil 3 or 4 minutes each side, or until juices run clear. Serve.

SAGE AND GARLIC PORK

1 tablespoon sage leaves, roughly torn
1 clove garlic, minced
Sea salt and freshly ground black pepper, to taste
1 teaspoon extra-virgin olive oil
One 4-ounce bone-in pork chop

In a bowl, combine the sage, garlic, salt, pepper, and oil. Add the pork and thoroughly coat. Marinate for 10 minutes.

In a nonstick sauté pan over medium heat, cook the pork for 3 to 4 minutes on each side, then cover with a lid. Serve with cauliflower "mashed potatoes" and a salad of mixed greens.

SOFT SCRAMBLED EGGS WITH CRUMBLED FETA, WILTED SPINACH, AND BABY TOMATOES

2 large eggs
Sea salt and freshly ground black pepper, to taste
½ tablespoon unsalted butter
¼ cup baby spinach leaves
¼ cup sliced baby yellow tomatoes
½ ounce crumbled feta cheese
½ tablespoon fresh chives, chopped (optional)

Whisk eggs and a sprinkling of sea salt and pepper in a medium bowl. Melt butter in a medium nonstick sauté pan over medium heat. When foam subsides, add eggs and stir with a heatproof spatula or wooden spoon for about 2 minutes, or until eggs are almost cooked but still runny in some places. Add the spinach, tomatoes, and feta, and cook for another 1 to 2 minutes. Remove from heat and serve, garnished with optional chives.

TEMPEH WITH BABY BOK CHOY AND MUNG BEAN SPROUTS

One 4-ounce piece tempeh, sliced into ¼-inch slabs
3 teaspoons sesame oil, divided
Juice of ½ lemon
⅛ teaspoon fresh or dried thyme
⅛ teaspoon garlic powder
Sea salt and freshly ground black pepper, to taste
1 clove garlic, minced
1 head baby bok choy, cut into eighths with some core still
    attached
1 teaspoon fresh ginger, grated
2 to 3 tablespoons low-sodium vegetable stock or water
½ cup mung bean sprouts

Preheat oven to 375° F. In a bowl, toss the tempeh with 1 teaspoon of the sesame oil, and the lemon juice, thyme, garlic powder, salt, and pepper. Spread the tempeh in a single layer on a baking sheet and bake for 15 to 20 minutes, or until lightly golden, flipping them halfway through.

While the tempeh is baking, warm 2 teaspoons of oil in a sauté pan over medium heat. Add the garlic and sauté about 15 seconds, until fragrant. Add the bok choy, ginger, and vegetable stock and cook about 3 minutes, or until bok choy is tender. Add the mung bean sprouts and sauté another 1 to 2 minutes. To serve, arrange greens and sprouts and top with tempeh.

WHITE BALSAMIC VINAIGRETTE

¼ teaspoon Dijon mustard
½ tablespoon white balsamic vinegar
¼ shallot, minced
Sea salt and freshly ground black pepper, to taste
2 tablespoons extra-virgin olive oil

In a small bowl, whisk together the mustard, vinegar, shallot, salt, and pepper. While whisking, slowly add the olive oil in a steady stream. Taste for seasoning and serve.

The No-Weight Workout

I developed the no-weight workout with the help of Bryant Stiney, a terrific trainer and change maker in his own right. Bryant developed the movement and exercise program at Shades of Hope Treatment Center in Buffalo Gap, Texas, and you will see him on the upcoming show on the Oprah Winfrey Network I have been involved with. He is also in the videos we have online at *JUST10Challenge.com* to help you get started with yoga and other no-weight workouts.

The no-weight workout is based on the principle that with the addition of just one simple piece of equipment and the use of your own body weight, you can change your workouts significantly and challenge your muscles to achieve the results you want. This is where "glider discs" enter your home gym.

Used widely in gyms today, glider discs resemble Frisbees. You place your feet on them to do a variety of effective toning exercises. You can use a hand towel in place of the glider.

Glider discs are an amazing tool—they're inexpensive, portable, and can be used to strengthen your whole body. Many exercises using these discs challenge your levels of speed and power and allow you to do many moves that are often difficult when using traditional strength-training equipment. The following warm-ups and five exercises work with any fitness level.

Warm-up

Warm up for 5 to 10 minutes with cardio (jogging lightly in place, jumping jacks, walking up and down stairs, and stretching your hamstrings and quadriceps).

Sliding Warm-up

Place one foot on each disc or hand towel. The point is to provide a way for each foot to "glide" effortlessly on the wood, tile, or linoleum floor. Bend over and hold on to a sturdy chair or bench for support. Slide your feet back and forth in an alternating fashion.

Sliding Lunges

Stand with your feet hip-width apart, hands on your hips, toe of the left foot resting on the disc. Bend your right leg while sliding the left foot back into a lunge position, keeping your right knee behind the toe, torso upright, and abs in. Slowly slide your left foot back to starting position and repeat for three sets of 12 repetitions on each side.

Chair Squats

Stand in front of a sturdy chair with your feet hip-width apart, abs tight and "in," and back straight. Slowly bend your knees and lower until you're almost touching your butt to the chair. Hold for 2 to 3 seconds. Keep your knees aligned behind the toes, and straighten up. Repeat for three sets of 12 repetitions.

Ab Slides

Begin in a push-up position, but on your knees, hands directly below your shoulders and resting on the discs or hand towels. Contract your abs and very slowly slide your hands straight out in front of you. Only go as far as you can without straining your back. Slide back to start and repeat for three sets of 12 repetitions.

Hamstring Slides

Lie down on your back with your knees bent and one disc or hand towel under your right foot. Lift your hips off the floor into a bridge position (commonly used in pilates and yoga). Press into the floor and slide your right foot out in front of you. Contract your hamstring and continue pressing into the floor as you slide the right foot back to starting position. Repeat for three sets of 12 repetitions on each side.

Glute Squeeze

Lie down on your back on an exercise mat or carpet with your knees bent. Lift your hips off the floor into a bridge position. Move your right leg straight into the air. Then lower your entire back down to the floor. Repeat for three sets of 12 repetitions on each side.

Family-Mapping Legends

Family-Mapping Legend

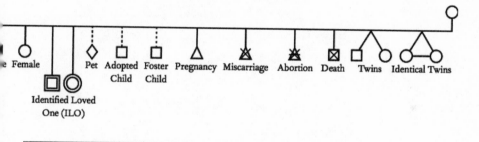

Female · Pet · Adopted Child · Foster Child · Pregnancy · Miscarriage · Abortion · Death · Twins · Identical Twins

Identified Loved One (ILO)

Family-Relationship Legend

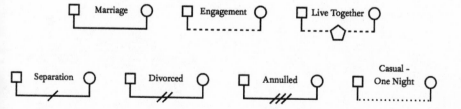

Marriage · Engagement · Live Together

Separation · Divorced · Annulled · Casual – One Night

About the Author

Brad Lamm is an author and educator best known for helping people make life-enhancing change on *The Dr. OZ Show.*

Brad is the founder of Intervention Specialists, a crisis intervention group helping family and friends enable a resistant loved one to make changes using his "invitational" intervention method whereby the loved one is invited to his or her own intervention. In 2008, Brad founded Change Institute to help inform and inspire folks to live better, lighter lives through weight loss and smoking cessation programs.

Brad believes that one's circle of friends and family is uniquely poised to offer support, accountability, and structure from a beginning point of love and honesty—no matter how broken-down or discouraged they may feel.

Highly motivated and with a history of long-term recovery himself, Brad has a teaching style that is no-nonsense and accessible, blending hope with the dynamic nature of his work. Previously a network-affiliate news anchor, his TV work today centers on his role as a regular on *The Dr. OZ Show.* He is a creator and producer of an upcoming series for OWN (The Oprah Winfrey Network).

Visit Brad at *www.Just10Challenge.com* and *www.ChangeInstitute. com.*

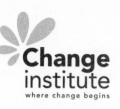

Change
institute
where change begins

About Change Institute

"I founded Change Institute to offer education, systems, and support to those seeking to live better, healthier lives. There's not just one way to change, and so we explore different paths and processes to equip you to live life brilliantly."
— BRAD LAMM

Visit *www.ChangeInstitute.com* for Brad's Invitation to Change Weight + Food Coaching Program and your free consultation with one of our Invitation to Change coaches.

Call our helpline at 1-800-818-0372 or register online now.

Our 90-Day Food + Weight Coaching Program includes:

- Weekly telephone and online support meetings

- Change agreements and goal coaching

- Spirit development coaching

NOTES

NOTES

Hay House Titles of Related Interest

YOU CAN HEAL YOUR LIFE, the movie,
starring Louise L. Hay & Friends
(available as a 1-DVD program and an expanded 2-DVD set)
Watch the trailer at: **www.LouiseHayMovie.com**

THE SHIFT, the movie,
starring Dr. Wayne W. Dyer
(available as a 1-DVD program and an expanded 2-DVD set)
Watch the trailer at: **www.DyerMovie.com**

✦

THE CORE BALANCE DIET: 4 Weeks to Boost Your
Metabolism and Lose Weight for Good,
by Marcelle Pick, MSN, OB/GYN NP

A COURSE IN WEIGHT LOSS: 21 Spiritual Lessons for
Surrendering Your Weight Forever, by Marianne Williamson

THE SPARK: The 28-Day Breakthrough Plan for
Losing Weight, Getting Fit, and Transforming Your Life,
by Chris Downie

✦

All of the above are available at your local bookstore,
or may be ordered by contacting Hay House (see next page).

✦

We hope you enjoyed this Hay House book. If you'd like to receive our online catalog featuring additional information on Hay House books and products, or if you'd like to find out more about the Hay Foundation, please contact:

Hay House, Inc., P.O. Box 5100, Carlsbad, CA 92018-5100
(760) 431-7695 or (800) 654-5126
(760) 431-6948 (fax) or (800) 650-5115 (fax)
www.hayhouse.com® • **www.hayfoundation.org**

✦

Published and distributed in Australia by: Hay House Australia Pty. Ltd., 18/36 Ralph St., Alexandria NSW 2015 • Phone: 612-9669-4299 Fax: 612-9669-4144 • www.hayhouse.com.au

Published and distributed in the United Kingdom by: Hay House UK, Ltd., 292B Kensal Rd., London W10 5BE • Phone: 44-20-8962-1230 Fax: 44-20-8962-1239 • www.hayhouse.co.uk

Published and distributed in the Republic of South Africa by: Hay House SA (Pty), Ltd., P.O. Box 990, Witkoppen 2068 • *Phone/Fax:* 27-11-467-8904 www.hayhouse.co.za

Published in India by: Hay House Publishers India, Muskaan Complex, Plot No. 3, B-2, Vasant Kunj, New Delhi 110 070 • *Phone:* 91-11-4176-1620 *Fax:* 91-11-4176-1630 • www.hayhouse.co.in

Distributed in Canada by: Raincoast, 9050 Shaughnessy St., Vancouver, B.C. V6P 6E5 • *Phone:* (604) 323-7100 • *Fax:* (604) 323-2600 • www.raincoast.com

✦

Take Your Soul on a Vacation

Visit **www.HealYourLife.com**® to regroup, recharge, and reconnect with your own magnificence. Featuring blogs, mind-body-spirit news, and life-changing wisdom from Louise Hay and friends.

Visit **www.HealYourLife.com** today!

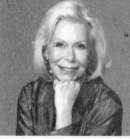
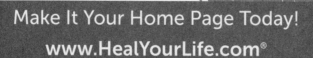